Walking on Jupiter

Andy Elliott

Walking on Jupiter

(Working against the planet in a good way)

Disclaimer:

The author Andy Elliott is not a licenced or a qualified physical trainer or instructor but has rather gained knowledge and experience of exercise and its effect on the body through many years of study.

Before commencing any exercise program, it is highly recommended that you consult with a doctor or medical expert to ensure that you are well and able to carry out the exercises recommended in this book.

It is my own personal belief that the exercise contained in this book, "Walking on Jupiter," are simple exercises that can be done by the majority of people with minimal risk of injury.

Please be aware that if you are carrying out the recommendations in this book then it is at your own risk and the author Andy Elliott will not be responsible or liable to any injury or harm that you may sustain whilst carrying out these exercises.

All exercises are recommendations only by the author and any person carrying out these exercises are free to alternate or vary from the suggested exercises or routines.

Any data contained in this book for examples weight, calories etc are not precise figures but can vary according to the individual.

It is the responsibility of the participant to ensure that they work in a safe environment using solid and sturdy fixings should they need these for support.

Walking on Jupiter
(Working against the planet in a good way)

Ever wanted that wonderful physique, despite age or current physical condition, but couldn't face going to the gym?
Ever wanted to be liberated from a strict exercise and diet regime?

With Walking on Jupiter, you will require: -
No visits to the Gym
No Dumbbells or Barbells
No Keep Fit equipment
No special diet or expensive supplements
No fixed number of sets, repetitions, and workouts
No repetitive routines week after week
No jogging for miles to lose weight

If all that sounds good to you, then get ready for: -

Walking on Jupiter

Table of Contents

Page

Walking on Jupiter – Really!!!

I know, I know; No one can really walk on Jupiter. Even if you wore the right space suit and had all the right equipment, it would still be impossible; Why? Because the planet is one huge ball of gas, made up primarily of hydrogen, and we all know that we can walk in gas but not on gas.
The title of this book is purely hypothetical, a means to an end.
It describes a new method of exercise which you will discover later in this book.
A format of exercise that offers great results by copying, yes copying the effects of the exercises that can be done at the gym such as the Bench Press, Curls, Shrugs, Shoulder Press, Rowing, to name but a few. However, you won't be lifting any physical weights. Your mind will just think that you are.
May sound a little wacky now, but it will become clearer a little later on.

To explain a little further, let's go back to the largest planet in our Solar System, Jupiter.
If the mass of Jupiter was made up of a solid structure such as planet Earth is, then yes, we could in theory walk on Jupiter. However, because of the great mass of the planet being around 1,300 times greater than Earth, the ability to do anything on this great planet would be so much harder due to the strong gravitational pull.
Imagine the effort therefore of simply going up stairs carrying many times your body weight? It would be like someone above you pushing down on your shoulders making the stair walk far more difficult. You may do it, but it would be very hard.
Let's apply that same principle to exercise. Imagine if you will that you are lifting or pushing a weight and going through all the motions including the tensing of the muscle as you go from point A to point B of the movement.
The body would have to react to the tension applied to it. How does it react?
Initially your body would tire very quickly, just as though you were physically lifting weights in the gym. The long-term effects would be: Burning more calories, toning, shaping, and making the muscles stronger. For every action, there is a reaction.

You are about to create the body that you really want rather than the one that has just evolved by your natural everyday living and ageing process.
Up to this point in your life, things may have just happened without you giving any rational thought about why you are what you are.
Even if you have exercised before, have you ever stopped to consider why you are doing what you are doing and is what I'm doing really going to benefit me?

If you follow just some of the principles in this book you will start to create a new you. Not just going through the motions of an exercise program such as 1 Press Up, 2 Press Ups……………now I've got to 10 Press Ups. Press Ups now completed. Just what the magazine article stated. Job done.
No. From now on you are going to make every movement count. Not only in a physical way but also in a mindful way. In other words, no part of the exercise will be wasted.
Whether you are using the WOJ (Walking on Jupiter) method or the more traditional body weight resistance exercises, also explained in this book, each movement will be of tremendous benefit to you, to help you achieve your physical goal.

I'm really excited to tell you about both forms of exercises later in this book, but for now I had better offer you the…………

Introduction – The dumb factor

I suppose it all started about 2 years ago. Up to that point, I, like most other people who exercised, tried to commit to regular training patterns. You know what I mean? I must train at 6:30 a.m. every Monday, Wednesday, and Friday. If I miss a workout, I will feel guilty and I expect my body to suddenly go back to how it was before I even started to exercise, just because I missed one workout.

I tried again and again, only to embrace the same frustration and disappointments, because of my missed exercise routines. I followed a delusional thought pattern of, "My body is never going to change if I only do two workouts this week instead of three." I would therefore yoyo back and forth working out with a feeling of obligation instead of heading towards any particular physique goal.

Added to this, I also thought that completing a certain number of repetitions and sets was absolute key to that better body. Why? Simply because I used to read all the latest physique training books and magazines.
If the top Pro's did 8 reps for 10 sets to build bigger arms, then that's what I must do to build bigger arms, right? If I only managed 9 sets instead of 10, then I've blown it. "Now I'm never going to add more muscle!" Not only did that not work, I realised that I was taking advice from someone who was probably a genetic superman, who most likely took steroids, was ripped a week prior to a big bodybuilding competition, wore a fake tan and was covered from head to toe in baby oil!
That's not me and I'm sure that's not you. We live in the real world!

The best equipment syndrome! Yes, I've been there and done that. Bought the latest shiny dumbbell set and gone to the gyms with the newest equipment thinking that my results were dependent upon the machines instead of man! I used to watch those exercise equipment commercials and naturally thought that if they look that good from that piece of equipment then the equipment must be the answer. Wrong again. It only took me around 45 years to discover that the best piece of equipment was me.

At the end of the day the body only changes according to the demands placed upon it physically and mentally and not how new and finely crafted the machine is.

As you can imagine, frustration set in quite quickly again when I wasn't achieving anywhere near the look, I set out to achieve. So, I started the blame game. It's the routine I'm doing! Or these top ten tips from Mr. Pro bodybuilder and all the latest scientific breakthroughs just doesn't work for me. Or these latest DVD's on, "How to get a Mr. Universe body in just 6 weeks." are faulty!
However, out of respect, there are a lot of trainers, coaches, and physique experts out there who do know what they are doing and have contributed a lot to the world of physical development.
If you want to get a physical trainer then fine, just make sure you get the right one. The one who's been through the blood, sweat and tears. Who's persevered, who's got the look, the knowledge and the know how to help you on your journey to that better body.

I also went down the road of super supplements. I naturally thought, that if I took this latest muscle mass gain powder, mix it with milk and drink two pints of it a day I too would achieve a Mr. Wonderful physique in next to no time. After all, it works for the guy in the picture, right?
Don't get me wrong, I did get bigger, but all of it round the waist and double the amount of time on the toilet! What I didn't realise was that the stars in these magazines were most likely paid very well for endorsing the latest powders and potions, scientifically designed to get you the ultimate body in 30 days or less!

Today we have multimedia devices so that we can watch the guys and the gals with the toned body, and hey what's that, "We can buy your latest super ripped DVD set at fifty percent discount if we are one of the first one hundred subscribers. Wow! Where's my credit card?"
Please forgive my sarcasm. I do need to point out that not all routines, equipment, and supplements are bad. What I'm trying to point out is; don't be misled into spending a lot of time and money on purchasing the magic pills of

success, that if you take it, your whole body will be transformed. It's not going to happen.
Be prepared to be in it for the long haul. It will happen, but not overnight!

When your body does change it will often be in sporadic bursts and not linear. That is why a lot of the time you will exercise and see little or no gains. That is when a lot of people give up and say, "I've tried exercising but it just doesn't work for me. I must have a body that is just fat!"

There is no such thing as the perfect, routine, food, supplement, or piece of equipment. My body, and your body is constantly changing and as I'll explain later it gets used to what exercises you are doing very quickly to try and maintain the status quo. In other words, our bodies will do their very best to remain constant and you sometimes must fight for the changes that you want.

So, who am I? My name is Andy Elliott and I have had a passion for exercise and physical development for around 50 years. Why? Because a friend of mine called Ian once laughed at my stick like arms when I was around 10 years of age. It's amazing what a little intimidation can do! Looking back, my arms were as big as my wrists are now and I still have small wrists! From that moment on, I read about more than I exercised about what to do to beef up.
As I grew and started to gather weight on the waist, I thought it's about time I put all this theory into practice. The mathematicians amongst us will have worked out that I'm now 60 years old and am still passionate about exercise. However, after trying out virtually every training system under the sun, I wanted to break away from the standard number of reps, sets and training days.

Most people don't have the time, inclination or maybe even the money for gym membership and so also want to be liberated from all of this, "Set routine stuff."
The how is, is easy. It's the doing it that requires hard work, dedication, and commitment.
So now I'll tell you what I don't do and in the following pages tell you what I do, do.

So here's my no, no list.....................................

No particular number of reps, or training sets.
No just going through the motions of exercise. Each repetition should be a master class of movement to fully achieve maximum muscular benefit.
No set days for workouts.
No training at a gym (but you can if you want to).
No special diet or supplements.
No artificial substances such as growth hormones, pills, or potions.
No special equipment, but a kitchen unit or chair can come in useful for Body Weight exercises.
No Sit Ups.
No special clothing.
No dedicated aerobic type exercises such as jogging, exercise bike etc.
No (Okay, very little actually) isolated exercises. Prefer compound movements. (Explain later).
In fact, NO set anything.

Sounds liberating, doesn't it?

Don't like doing things in a set order? Then why not do ....

Just Random Acts of Exercise

If you are currently very much out of shape and the thought of going to a gym terrifies you, then hopefully my no, no list will have encouraged you to read on.

Total flexibility that allows you to exercise when and where you like. Hence the title of this chapter. No fixed rules that dictate where, when and what you should do.
No need to carry a set of dumbbells around with you in your handbag!
Just random. Do just one exercise if you have a spare couple of minutes or maybe 10 exercises if you have half an hour.
The choice is yours. No excuses please?

Often, that's what kills it in the first place. Many people think that in order to get into great shape they either have to go jogging because they see lots of Joggers out there or they have to go to a gym or Fitness Club.
Added to that that they think that they have to spend a lot of money in having a personal trainer, which seems to be the trend these days. No problem in that. However, if they have the mindset, which states that they are a 20 stone piece of overweight human being then the last thing they are going to want to be is embarrassed or humiliated. Thus, they don't go out at all and end up eating more because of their depressive state and then the downward spiral begins.
If that's you, then this book is for you.

What about my age?
Think you're too old, too out of shape, out of inspiration, out of hope, out of energy, to think that you can still have a great physique?
Do you think that you're past it and can no longer offer anything to yourself or society that will make any difference? Then please think again. It's time for a new mind shift.

These words are from the Old Testament in the Bible.

"Now then, just as the Lord promised, he has kept me alive for forty-five years since the time he said this to Moses, while Israel moved about in the wilderness. So here I am today, eighty-five years old (*YES, EIGHTY-FIVE YEARS OLD*). <u>I am still as strong today as the day Moses sent me out; I'm as vigorous to go out to battle now as I was then.</u> Now give me this hill country that the Lord promised me that day. You yourself heard then that the Anakites were there, and their cities were large and fortified, but the Lord helping me, I will drive them out just as he said."
Joshua 14: 10-12.

I'm not going to preach you a sermon, but I will say that if a man in his mid-eighties is ready to climb hills and do battles, what's your excuse?

Convinced? I hope you are because in a relatively small amount of time your body will change and so will your mind.
You will start to look forward to going out. You will be encouraged and strengthened from the inside out. The better the inside the better the outside.

In the opening chapters you will find out that the first exercise to do is not the body but rather the mind. If the mind isn't right the body will not follow. This isn't deep meditative stuff that involves going into some hypnotic trance but rather very simple internal changes that has a huge outcome on the outward physical changes.
The mind is where the blueprint is of how you want to be. Get the mind right and the body will certainly follow.

Coming up is................

A small section for the ladies

I read a report over a decade ago, which certainly applies today, maybe even more so.

A popular magazine did a poll of over 5,000 women and found that just one in fifty was happy with the way their body looked.

70% of women said their lives would improve if they had better bodies.

Illnesses such as bulimia and anorexia start with the thoughts of a distorted body image.

British women worry about their body once every fifteen minutes.

Virtually all women said that they have tried dieting at some point in their life.

Over 40% constantly watch what they ate.

Half admitted to lying about their weight.

Almost one third cut label sizes out of their clothes.

Most hated body part was thighs followed closely by the waist.

I'm guessing that if you are a lady reading the above then you can certainly relate to most of the above statements.
If you are looking for the perfect body, it's not going to happen because there is always going to be certain aspects of what and who you are that is not going to measure up to the ideal you. This, you will have to learn to live with.
However, you can learn to be far happier and more confident by having lots of small incremental changes in how you look and feel.

Reading and following the advice in this book will help you get nearer to that goal.

Someone once said, "You cannot pay someone to do the Press Ups for you." In other words, I can offer the instructions, but the physical and mental work will all be done by you.

A kite will only fly high when it works against the wind. If you want to soar, then you are going to have to work against the natural instinct of always wanting to be comfortable.
It's hard I know; but so is the disappointment of simply being in the same place in twelve months' time and saying to yourself, "If only?"
This is not a put down but rather an encouragement for what you can become over the coming weeks, months, and years.

We now live in an era where the ladies of this world are becoming more and more dependent upon themselves to get things done.
Why? Because there are a lot more weaker men out there who aren't getting the things done that should be done. Not just on a physical level in the terms of muscular development but at the workplace and in the home.
It's far easier to pass the buck, by saying, "It's not my job, I'm tired, I've had a hard day, stop nagging, I just want to watch TV."
Even in the workplace. Some will say I don't want a promotion, I'm happy to stay as I am. I want to be with my mates. We have a laugh.
Well guys it is time to, "Man up," to show them that you are the man that they love to be with. The Man that will watch over them, protect them, love them, and support them.

I love the Church that I go to. At the time of writing this book, church was a rented school hall and we had to set up each week with large boards that formed a backdrop to the worship group. It was some of the men that were saying, "Uh, I can't move those boards I have a bad back." It was the ladies that were saying, "Okay, we'll do it." I'm sorry, but I found that somewhat embarrassing.
Ladies tell your men, it time for them to be the men that God created them to be.

"Male by birth, but a man through choice."

There are now far more successful businesswomen who are entrepreneurs than ever before because they now have stronger beliefs of who they can become and what they can achieve.
Background, upbringing, race, genetics are no longer relevant to what you can become, both inside and out.

I know that there are a lot of very independent ladies out there and whether they choose to admit it, they are often that way because they have been let down by us guys. In some cases, so many times that they just give up on the men and have chosen a more independent life.

Remember, the new you is already in you. It's in your potential, your dreams, your passions, and your desires of how you want to be.
Let your imagination run wild. If you could be the person, you really wanted to be then realise that if you can think it, you can be it. However, the "Be it," comes with consistent action on a daily basis. Little and often until it becomes a regular part of you.
Your journey has already begun simply by reading this book. This is your first step.

Please don't think I am being chauvinistic, when I say, I'm not really into this Girl Power thing that was very prevalent a few years ago.
I'm simply saying that in my opinion, you too have been created to be the best that you can be. You have it within you and through a slow but consistent change in daily habits in the form of exercising, thoughts, words, actions, and your spiritual life you can change immensely into the person you want to be.

So, to the guys reading this, please don't think that I am putting the male species down. Quite the contrary. Men too must rise up and wise up and be the men they have to be. That means on every level.
Caring, compassionate, loving, generous, provider, attentive, romantic, reliable, strong, muscular, protector, confident. You don't have to be the most handsome guy on the planet. Just one that they can turn to and know that they are looked after on every level from the man in their life.

Deep down ladies isn't that the kind of man that you want in your life?

I mentioned in this chapter the word, "Spiritual." If you find this little word a bit spooky and is this Andy guy a bit wacky then please let me explain my beliefs in the next short chapter.

This is someone I met when I was 26 years of age. Gave my life to Him and never looked back. This is ....

The God Factor – In His image

So, what does God have to do with my physical wellbeing? Well, if you believe
that He created you, then it has everything to do with your wellbeing. As
human beings we are His highest form of creation.
In the first book of the bible (Genesis) God says, "Let us make man in Our
image." Also, just look at what our bodies can do and you will see that we are
no fluke or random act of chance.

Remember as a young child when you would colour a picture or make
something creative out of a few strips of cardboard. Or maybe you spent hours
producing something out of little plastic building bricks and then showed it to
your parents and then wait for what is hopefully a happy reaction.
Or maybe after many days, you finally finished a 1,000 pcs jigsaw. Do you just
break it all up straight after completing it? No, you want to show people,
because inwardly you're saying, look what I've done. Please be happy with me
and for me. It's a bonding thing. They're happy with you and what you have
achieved and that increases your happiness with them. A strengthening of
relationships.
Well it's the same with God. He created you, and He wants to say, "Look what I
have done." He's just so pleased and happy with you and He wants you to be
the same with Him.

Since He created me, I just feel that it's good to look after the body that He has
blessed me with and that is why I exercise to look after what He has given. To
me it's just natural. Take care of what has been gifted to you.

Am I therefore going to strive be perfect? No. Absolutely not. No one can reach
perfection. Rather I just aim to simply be the best that I can be whilst still being
a normal guy. No pressure.

So, a little more about God.
I need to point that when discussing spiritual and religious content it can be a
very touchy subject to a lot of people. I certainly don't mean to offend anyone.
I believe that God gave us free will to choose and I chose Him.

There are a huge number of different beliefs out there relating to the word, "Spiritual." From all the different religions in the world to different forms of meditation found in various forms such as Yoga.
What's more, we all think that our way is the right way and often the only way!

Mine is very simple. I don't lose myself in the cosmos, I don't go into meditative trances or chant mantras so that the universe can hear me and provide my needs. I don't burn scented candles so that I can get lost in the aroma's and I never empty my mind. If I do that who knows not what will come in and occupy that void?
I don't mess with tarot cards or try to talk to the other side. I don't mess with crystals, and I certainly do not hug trees!

I am simply a Christian. So, what does that mean?
It means that I have given my life and trust in Jesus Christ who is the Son of God. I constantly repent of my sins, and I believe that He died on the cross for me and all of mankind to take away our sins. On the third day after He died God raised Him up from the dead and now, He dwells in Heaven with His Father.
Why, did He choose to die? He did it for us, so that we can have a relationship with God through His son, Jesus.
That's it in its simplest form.

It's also about relationship. To know that God is watching over me, taking care of me through every situation. Guiding me through life.
Sure, we all have friends and families, but are they always there 24/7? Are they 100% reliable? Can they always give you the correct answers in life? Can they love you so much that they will die for you? Can they always forgive you and take away your sins, heal your wounds, provide your needs?
My God can, through Jesus Christ His Son. At 26 years of age I gave my life to Him and never looked back.
Being a Christian isn't always easy. But for me is worth it.

My question for you is, What or who do you have faith in?
Your life. Your choice.

Off course, I have done and will continue to face hardships and unpleasant situations, but I have Him there with me helping me and strengthening me through those times.

For me, knowing Jesus has made me content. I am satisfied with who I am. I no longer have to try and achieve lots of things to try and win peoples approval or get them to like me. I don't have to be the most popular guy on the planet. I am content.

That doesn't mean I still don't want to improve the things in my life. Of course I do and so should you. However, please be content with every stage of your life and don't get caught in the trap of trying to get people to like you 100% of the time. It's not going to happen. Going down that road can take you into the realms of depression, anxiety, hurt, shame to name but a few.

If that is you start shouting it out now, "I am content." Love yourself because the God of Love made you. Be satisfied with what He made.

I can't force you to know God through His son Jesus, but for me, it's the best choice I ever made. In fact, it's an eternal choice.

You can believe in nothing and take your chance in life and yes you may have been dealt a good hand and live a pretty good, healthy, and prosperous life. You may live well into your nineties and die. But is that it?

After all I believe that the decision of accepting Jesus Christ as the Lord of your life determines where you will be for all of eternity.

I'll say it again, "Your life, your choice."

Why not live a life of purpose? I believe that God gave me a purpose in writing this book so that you can read this chapter and make your own choice, with your own free will.

I said this was a small chapter and I could write page after page about my belief in God, but It is not my intention to take it much further in this book.

All I will say is, that if you want to know more, then get along to a good Bible believing Church and speak to the Pastor or any Christians that you know and trust. I'm sure they will be willing to help.

Now, you know what…………………

I've changed my mind – Good

Most of us have probably said at some point in our lives, "I've changed my mind." That means we're either doing something or about to do something but then something happened to cause you to, "Change your mind." We then went in a different direction and achieved a different set of results.
We sometimes say that sheep are not the brightest of animals. When several people do the same dumb thing, we say, "They're just like sheep following each other around. Doing one dumb thing after another."

Have you ever questioned why you do what you do? Even when doing what you do, doesn't get you the results that you want. However, instead of changing, we carry on doing the same things for weeks and sometimes even years on end, even if no beneficial results are apparent.
It's simply called, "Habit." We're so wired into our own internal hard drive that we have to do as our neurological pattern tells us. If we deviate from what we normally do, a few days later, we're back doing the same old thing. Crazy, but true!
It's basically down to our internal defence mechanism. Our body will do all that it can to protect itself. A change in habits could prove dangerous, therefore do what you have always done and stay comfortable, is what our mind is telling us to do.
That is why New Year resolutions rarely work. Remember all those good intentions you had of losing weight, getting fitter, gym membership, looking for a new job? Those thoughts you had at the beginning of the Year? Where are those dreams now?

However, you may be the exception to the rule. You may be reading this right now and getting all enthusiastic. "Yes, I am going to change, I am going to do it. The new me is about to emerge. I am going on that diet, and I am going to lose five stone and I am going to look good on the beach this year. I am going to tell my boss what they can do with their job!" Really?
The trouble with enthusiasm and motivation is that they never seem to be there when you need them. Thus, you very often fail to see things through

because your internal wiring takes you right back to your starting point and the comfort of your comfort zone.

So, if you want to break with convention and achieve a different set of results, you have to change your mind in a very strong and compelling way. You may have to break free of the herd and find a new field to graze in. One that will make you flourish. It's not easy to do. In fact, it's incredibly hard to do, but with massive and consistent action it can be done, and I believe in you to do it.

Experts tell us that it takes around 30 to 40 days to form a new long-lasting habit. Trouble is it takes a lot of effort to go those 30 days in the first place to form that new habit.

To do so you must have an end result in mind and a desire so strong that you are compelled to do whatever it takes.

How many times have you said, "I should this and I should that, and if I want to improve then I should do, whatever?" Should is a weak word, and should, should be replaced with a must. A must is a very compelling and strengthening word. A must is a call to immediate action to get things done.

As this book is primarily about getting a great physical body, let's look for a moment about how changing your mind will take you one step further towards that goal.

Most people who are dissatisfied with their bodies will look at themselves in the mirror and their pre-programmed mind will tell them everything that's wrong with them from flabby arms, bulbous waistlines, large hips, saggy pecs, drooping shoulders and so on.

Their mind will also tell them, that you were just made that way. It's in the genes and there is nothing you can do about it. Just accept it. Why? Because the body doesn't want to do a workout! It doesn't want to change its diet of chocolate and chips. It just wants the easy life of keeping things as they are.

So, within just seconds you can literally talk yourself out of taking any action.

However, if you can talk yourself out of it, then you can also talk yourself into it.

The power of two

It's a little like a seesaw that you used to see in a lot of playgrounds. If you constantly have negative thoughts, actions, and words then the results will all be one-sided. In this case the bad side.

However, let's suppose that you have a friend standing near the other side of the of see-saw and is a very positive influencer. That person will tell you that everything is possible. You can get into great shape, you can change your eating habits, you can walk more, exercise more and what's more I am going to help you. I will encourage you and make you accountable to me.

Now you have options. Are you going to listen to yourself or to your positive influencer?

You're reading this book because you do want change. So, my guess is that you are going to listen to someone who is going to help and not hinder you.

That person now gets on the see-saw who is slightly heavier than you (in a muscular way of course!) and so as you feel a little more elated and physically elevated you would automatically lean towards that positive person as the seesaw rises.

Together, as the power of two. Change starts to happen.

Faith is stronger than fact. Your changed mind must see things as you want them to be. Strong, toned arms. A slim waistline, even with hints of a six pack. Slimmer hips. Defined pectorals. Strong broad shoulders.

A changed mind will take a step of courage and say enough is enough, the time has come, and the time is now.

To see yourself in your mind's eye of how you want to be and how you want to look and how you want to feel.

Even as you are reading this, your whole being should be sensing a change. You feel that passion rising up on the inside of how things are going to be from now on.

That passion is a call to action.

It makes you rise above all the disappointments of the past. The past is behind you, and you don't need to get it back to live in it anymore.

You can't change the past, but you can direct your future.

A changed mind leads to a good mind, which leads to a passionate mind, which leads to desires, which leads to that MUST and not a should.
If you have that MUST, then you have every reason to push forward because you've got conviction and if you have conviction then nothing is going to stop you from reaching your goals.

So now you have a solid conviction that change is going to happen.

The next thing you need to know is……………………

What do I want to look like, and do I have the desire to see it through?

Notice I said, "Look like." You use your mind to create an image. Forget about stones, and pounds, Kilo's and ounces. Forget about the numbers on a tape measure. Your mind can't equate the number 26" on a tape measure and relate it to what your waist will look like. Likewise, a 10 stone woman at 5 feet tall is going to look quite different to someone of the same weight at 5' 10". Your mind thinks and acts on pictures not on numbers.
If I were to say to you, "I am going to give you one million pounds," you wouldn't think of a number 1 followed by 6 zeros. No, you would think of all the wonderful things you could buy or give away with your one million pounds.

You must see in your own mind what you want to look like. See the waist you want to have, rather than what you have now. Be forward looking. After all, in life you are going forward into tomorrow, next week, next month and years to come. You cannot go back. So, set an image in your imagination of how you want to look now. The new ideal you.

Don't tell me that you don't know what you want to look like, yes you do. As you walk down the street, watch television, look at magazines, you're looking at other people all the time. Within a fraction of a second you mentally take in their body, their hair, their face, their clothes, their age, how they walk and if you're a woman, most likely their shoes!
You instantly make a judgement about that person and often about yourself. You do a mental comparison and decide whether you want to be more like them. If I had their figure, their hair etc then would I be happier?

You see we are always looking to find ways of being happier. You're naturally drawn to that feel-good factor and repel the things that will make you unhappy. It's inherent. It's the way we were created. We were made to constantly look forward to a better, brighter future. Sadly though we seldom step into that future but rather maintain the life we are comfortable in.
Are you really comfortable with the life you are in? Probably not, or else you wouldn't be reading this book, would you?

So, before we start Walking on Jupiter, I want you to spend some time on creating this image of the person you want to be.

Let's suppose a Carpenter is looking to make a new table, the first thing they are going to do is think about what the table is going to look like. After they have an image in mind they would probably draw the table with all the dimensions, wood type, finish etc.
The tools they have in the workshop will be used to cut, shape and mould the table until they are pleased with the end result. Along the way they may change the design slightly and that will in turn need more use of the tools. The end result however after many twists and turns along the way will bring forth the table.
So, create the image first. The exercises in the forthcoming pages are simply the tools required to mould and shape.

When creating an image, we will often imagine other people having what you want to have. That's fine. People use people all the time for inspiration. However, can I kindly ask you to never, never, never, idolise or worship another person. You are just as important as any other person on this planet. They may have a different figure to you, they may be more famous or have more money, but the bottom line is they are a human being just like you with equal rights on this planet.

Never beat yourself up because you are not like someone else. You are unique. You are special and not a clone of anyone else.

As I once heard someone say. "You make a lousy someone else, but a brilliant you."
So be inspired by others, learn from others, and be encouraged by others but do not treat them as idolised beings.

Now let's talk a little about love…………………………

Start to love yourself

Isn't that arrogant, boastful, and full of pride? Not if you do it right. If you start to brag about what you have achieved then yes, it is. If you go around just wanting to be noticed then yes, it is. Take my word for it, people do not like braggers. If what you do implies that you are better than someone else, then what you are saying is that, "I'm better than you." If you start to do that, you will soon become Little Billy no mates.

Not only that, but you will also be constantly battling others internally. Striving to outdo other people in every area you can think of. It's a battle that you will never win and will only lead to bitterness and frustration.

To "Love yourself," is to be pleased with who and what you are. If you constantly say things like, "I'm fat. I'll never be thin. Just look at the size of my thighs, I hate myself, it's not fair and why was I made this way?" Then you are on the way to worse, not better results. There's a verse in the Bible which says, "According to your faith, be it unto you." This means that whatever you say, particularly with belief and conviction then it will come to pass in your life.

If you say to yourself that I am fat, and with conviction believing it to be true enough times, guess what, you'll be fat. What's more it is you that bought it upon yourself because you had faith, even if it is negative faith, it is still faith. Through that faith you are programming your mind to hold on to additional fat. Your mind is not interested in whether or not you wanted that fat. Rather it is obeying your instructions to be fat. In other words, it is your fault.

Author, Earl Nightingale in his recording, "The Strangest Secret," Stated that we become what we think about most of the time.

Have you ever said, "I'm so tired, I'm exhausted, I can't go another step?" Then you get your body to follow through by flopping into a comfortable sofa whilst letting out a huge sigh so that everyone around you knows how really tired you are?

Notice I said flop into a sofa. Had you never said, "I'm exhausted", Then you probably would have just sat down quite normally. We follow through physically what our minds tell us to do.

I remember walking in the very picturesque Lake District in England. Travelling up a steep incline, I could feel my legs starting to ache and mentally I started saying to myself, "I'm getting tired. I must rest. I must find some excuse to stop and talk about the scenery." Then something clicked inside of me and instead, I said, "I've got Powerised Thighs." Over and over and within just a few seconds, I found a new energy that easily got me up to the top of that hill.
Remember that the mind will always give out before the body.

If you say, "Your fat," over and over again, it's simple, you'll be and stay fat, because that is your self-image and you will not find any enthusiasm to exercise. You will mentally draw upon literally hundreds of excuses of why you are not going to do it. You have just given your body a solid reason to stay fat. Equally, even if you are currently an overweight Blobbychops, (Yes, that is a made-up word) you can just as easily say, "Wow, I feel great. I've got energy. I am going to follow through. Fat, you're coming off and staying off."
Speak to yourself constantly. Picture yourself of how you want to look with confidence knowing that it is possible and very soon that new habit and thus the new you will start to emerge.

Now is the time to take responsibility for yourself and make a different decision that will bring the results that you do want in life. A new change of thought pattern that will bring you that new design of body that you want so badly.

Loving yourself is the key. Some people love their car. They wash it, polish it, vacuum it, and only drive it if the sun is shining. If they take that much care over a manmade vehicle, then surely you being a God made person is far more important. After all you must live with yourself every day. So, you may as well love yourself, whilst you live with yourself.

Your mind is the most important tool in your toolbox to restructuring you. Get this right and the rest will follow.

Changing your thoughts.
Rather than look at yourself in the mirror and think, oh no, I'm a 20-stone
disaster, think of yourself as that slender thing you want to be. Or maybe a
great muscular guy that you know is within you. Following are the tools to let
the new you come from the inside out.
The better images you can get in your mind of how you want to be then the
better the results because you are reprogramming your mind as to how you
want to look.

Spend a few minutes each day, visualising how the New You will look. How
would you describe yourself? If you're a man, you might think of some of those
guys from the action movies and picture yourself with those strong arms and a
six pack. You might see yourself with those broad shoulders and prominent
pecs.
Ladies, you may see yourself with that perfect hourglass figure.
Don't just see the pictures, rather see yourself as the starring role in the movie.
The guys might be doing some strongman act such as saving the damsel in
distress. See yourself running through the woods, jumping over roof tops,
climbing the cliff face. Can you see the peak on the biceps? Can you feel the
width of your back wanting to burst through your shirt? Are you sweating as
you arrive on the scene just in time? See it as though it is real.

You ladies might see yourself wearing that size 10 dress. Where are you
wearing it? In the office, in the park, at a party? Are all those people really
looking at me and thinking, "How did she get that figure? I only saw her a few
weeks ago. What a transformation!"
What's the weather like? Who's around you? What noises can you hear? The
stronger the emotional attachment the more real it becomes. The more real it
becomes the quicker your mind will tell the body; this is how it's supposed to
be. Make this a new habit. The more you project those images in the mind, the
easier it becomes, just like any other habit. You may see this as a silly exercise,
but it's powerful and its fun as you can be the person of your dreams.

Every day you fill your mind with so much information. Unfortunately, most of it is bad and depressing such as terrible news on the television, or gossip in the newspapers and magazines.

My advice would be to try and filter out those aspects of news that try and capture your attention. Those negative stories can, if you're not careful drag you down and have you feeling very sorry for yourself. However, as you read this, declare that this is a new day. A brand-new life, that's starting for you and in you today. You will be able to exercise so much better if you are full of joy. Your body was designed that way. The more upbeat you are, the healthier you become.

I recently read about a man in hospital who only had a 5% chance of living because of a serious illness. He thought well if I'm going to die, I may as well go out happy. So, from his bedside he watched continuously old Laurel and Hardy comedy films. As he did so his mind and body changed because of what was happening internally. In fact, he changed to such an extent that he beat his illness and lived. That's the power of a changed attitude.

Just as your body needs physical nourishment in the form of food and water your mind needs nourishment in the form of good thoughts, images, words, and emotions. Do this and within a short time you will be amazed at the difference.

Your mind is your mind. No one can change your mind except for you. You always have a choice. So, if you're going to change your mind, change it for good. Very soon if you apply yourself to the exercises laid out in the following pages, changes will occur if you stick with it.

Love is the strongest of all emotions. If a boy loves a girl, he'll walk over hot coals to get to her. He'll pull out all the stops just to be with her. The daydreaming begins. Loads of different scenarios will play upon his mind. His emotions run wild. He has a buzz of excitement welling up within him. His character changes. In fact, everything changes within him when he feels that he is in love.

The people he's with will also notice the changes. As the song goes, "That's the Power of Love."

It all starts in the mind. It's just bubbling up on the inside. Shake a bottle of pop or champagne and then release the cork and wow it just explodes, as the energy is released. Imagine if that is you just before a workout. How different would your exercise be.
Learn to love yourself. Irrespective of what you may look like right now. Irrespective of what your past has been like. You can't live there anymore. It's gone, it's happened. Only your future is yet untold and you're about to take your next step into it.

Love really does conquer all. I am not trying to hype you up or belittle sad situations that you may have been through in the past. I know of some people who have had terrible pasts.
It's hard I know, and some people can grieve for many years about what has happened to them or loved ones around them. What I am simply asking is that you give love and forgiveness a chance.

If you ask yourself a question, then your mind will have try and find a way of answering it.
It may give you many different answers. It is then up to you to filter out what is the right answer and the best long-term solution to your problem.

The following is a list of some good questions. Try asking yourself these and find out what can be done to make your life a whole lot better.

- Is it now time for me to move on?
- What small step can I take to making just one improvement in my life today?
- What can I be happy about right now?
- What am I thankful for (try and list at least 5 items)?
- Who can I show more love and appreciation too?
- Who can I forgive right now for a wrong that has been done towards me? (This applies to someone who is either alive or not).
- Who can I encourage?
- How can I reduce my calorie intake by just a small amount?
- What just one exercise could I do that will encourage me to do more?

- Can I just walk a little further tomorrow than I did today?
- What dreams that I once had can be rekindled?
- What is really stopping me from moving forward right now?

The list is basically endless and what you can do is limitless.
Maybe this is a good time to not read any further until you have done a little self-examination. Read through those questions again and if it helps to bury some of your past conflicts and helps you and others in the future then I'm really glad to have helped.

Now it's time to talk about exercise.

So…………

Why exercise and what are the benefits?

We all know that exercise is good for you. Benefits include weight loss (in the form of fat reduction), greater general health and fitness, increase in muscle mass, greater vitality and energy, a more pleasing body, to name but a few. However, there are many more reasons to exercise.

Here is some of the advantages of starting an exercise program.

- Reduced blood pressure
- Increased metabolism and therefore burn of fat more quickly
- Great antidepressant and therefore less stress
- Increases the quality of your sleep
- Lowers risk of cardiovascular disease such as heart attacks
- Reduces the effect of ageing
- Improves balance
- Slows down and can even reverse the decline in muscle mass, body strength and bone density. Usually considered irreversible in ageing
- Strengthens your immune system, therefore helping you to fight diseases
- Decreases appetite
- Strengthens your heart and lungs enabling you to work more efficiently
- Improves circulation and therefore supplies more oxygen to the brain helping you to think and reason
- One for the bosses – Less time off work for your employees if they are fitter, healthier, stronger and have renewed enthusiasm

Most of the above benefits relate to the physical you. However, there is a great mental advantage also. As you look and feel better on the outside you will feel improved on the inside. You will experience that inner joy and new-found confidence.

When you move with confidence, your shoulders are back, your chest is out, your breathing improves, your posture improves, your stride increases.

You'll also find that your thinking improves and your ability to move and do general tasks is far more increased.
You'll find that your life is starting to have more purpose.

Imagine yourself going out more and not being fearful that someone might comment on your weight or your overall look.
In fact, the reverse may be true. No, I don't mean that you will comment or be sarcastic about other people that you see. Rather, they will offer complimentary comments about how you have changed and how you now look and will be asking, "How on earth did you get into such great shape?"
How would you feel to be receiving those sorts of comments?

What's more, all the exercises you are about to discover can be done in the comfort of your own home. So, you can start today in making those improvements in your life.

Having read the above, you now know some of the benefits of exercise. At least in their basic form. However, laziness, procrastination, or a general I can't be bothered attitude, may have kept you from doing anything about it.
You may have said that, "Exercise is not for me. It doesn't rock my boat. I wouldn't know where to start. What's the point?"

May I ask you a question. "Deep, deep down, do you know that starting an exercise program is the right thing to do for you?" Take that question seriously and answer it seriously. I'm guessing that your answer is YES, or else you wouldn't be reading this book in the first place.
You know that you need to do something about your current condition both inside and out, because you know that you are more than you currently are.

If that is you then I thank-you for your honesty. If you stick with the exercises in this book you will change.

I can only put it down on paper, but you can make it happen.

Let's us now look at ……………

Exercise – A misunderstood word

Guess what? Did you know that you are exercising constantly? Each time you move a finger, turn your head, lift your hand to drink coffee, you are effectively using energy and therefore burning calories and therefore exercising. However, there is such a thing as effective or dedicated exercise. These times of course are when you are doing specific named exercises such as jogging, swimming, or getting down on the floor to do press ups. You are doing that particular movement for a reason.

A bodybuilder will do barbell curls to gain size, strength, and tone to his or her biceps. That is their specific reason for lifting that weight. As they lift, they are not thinking, this will really widen my back or make my calves bigger. No, because they are not exercising that body part. If they're good at what they do, they will put all their mental and physical effort into that movement to ensure that they receive the maximum benefit from that exercise to improve their arms.

This is not done by saying I've got to do 8 repetitions of this movement because the magazine article tells me to.
It's not done by following Mr Pro bodybuilder's routine. If they do it, I've got to do it, type attitude.
It's also not done because Miss Fitness model says in her DVD, just do what I do and you will lose 50 lbs of weight in just 4 weeks.
It's done by following your rules that you are going to lay out. Each exercise routine that you do should be fine-tuned to you, by you and nobody else. You do not have the mind or the body of someone else. You are uniquely you. What may be right for them, may not be right for you. Don't let anyone put you in a box and say you must do it this way. Consider this book as a guide. I believe it to be a good guide, but a guide nevertheless. If you want to go and choose a whole different way of doing exercise, then that's fine.

Let's say a pro-athlete has a benchmark number of repetitions that they are performing for chin ups. Normally they do 8 repetitions in good form. However today they are feeling very good about themselves. They feel that this is the day where they can achieve a personal best. They get mentally prepared and then go for it. 1,2,3,4,5,6,7,8,9 and yes, they just about squeeze out a 10th rep. They didn't say, "The article I read on chin ups told me only to do 8 reps, therefore I stopped at 8." No. They felt inside that today was the day. They knew that if they wanted to go to their next level of training and development they had to go all out. It was now or never.

If you are not a pro-athlete, then you probably won't do 8-10 chin-ups. If you're just starting out with exercising you may not even be able to do one. That's okay. You're unique. You may start with doing chin-ups whilst your feet are on a chair and thus pull up only part of your body weight. I still do that now, to concentrate on the muscles being contracted rather than the body weight I am lifting. Remember, don't lift other people's weights!
Do what you can do and do it well. Your body is remarkable. It will adapt very quickly to the demands you place upon it and your physique will change accordingly.

If you want to improve, you are going to have to have to toughen up your whole core and work against adversity, against the struggles, against the resistance.
Yes, it's hard, but that's where the rewards are.

A film where the hero simply walks into a castle, gets the princess and the treasure would be a little boring and would also be over in 5 minutes!
No, instead we're looking for our hero to fight overwhelming odds along the way. Winning battles and never giving up until he receives his prize.

Exercise. Yes, it is a misunderstood word. It can mean a walk to your kitchen cupboard to get a doughnut or a tough one-hour training session.
Again, it comes back to an individual you. It's what you make it.
Just beware of the mind, which always wants to take you upon the path of least resistance.

I hope that by now, you are encouraged to give this exercise thing a go. We are getting close, just a few more pointers to help you before you start.

Advisory points

I know you are probably eager to get going with the exercises but please be patient a little while longer and continue to read through these advisory points. They will be well worth it in the long run.

Where are you? I am making an assumption that you are training at home. You can of course do similar exercises at a gym which admittedly do have a wonderful assortment of equipment that can train virtually every part of your body.

The similarity is that any exercise equipment, no matter how high tech it is, will simply place resistance upon body parts which can be replicated by using your own body weight or even simply by flexing your muscles, which I will cover in more detail later.

As I explained in the Introduction of this book; you can of course pay for gym membership, and have an experienced trainer show you the equipment. They can show you how to do the exercises and advise on number of reps, sets and how often you should train. That's absolutely fine. No problem with that. That is the traditional way.

However, if you do not have the time, money or even the inclination to join the gym, that's also fine because using the WOJ method, you can do a set of exercise in the time it takes to put on your trainers to go to the gym.

In fact, in the time it takes to get to the gym you probably would have finished your workout using WOJ and it's FREE!

This method has great flexibility in that it can be used virtually anywhere and at any time.

In your home, at a hotel room, a caravan, a tent, even in your garden.

Be willing to be flexible. No exercise method needs to be written in stone!

We all know that there are literally hundreds of different exercises that we can do, some of course are much better than others. All exercises will have some effect on the body. What I'm now going to reveal is in my opinion some of the best exercises and how to perform them for maximum benefit. Starting with the mind preparation and working through to the completed set of exercise.

Firstly, I am going to go through the, "Walking on Jupiter," exercises. This basically replicates going to the gym. So, if anybody asks you where you go to exercise, you can tell them I visit a virtual gym! In the forthcoming chapters, I will explain about mindset, concentration, and the exercises. After that, I am going to go show you some more traditional exercises that I'm sure you have heard of but doing the exercises in a slow and controlled manner. Sounds a little wacky, but I'm sure that you will be impressed with the results.
The Virtual Gym exercises (WOJ) can be used either in conjunction with the body weight exercises or as a standalone type of exercise.
Remember, I am trying to offer you total liberation from set forms of exercise programs.
You don't need to go to a place to exercise. As the place is already right where you are wherever you are. You are the equipment!

Compound Exercises
These are movements which stimulate and effect several muscle groups at the same time. For example, when doing press ups, you are primarily working the pectoral muscles for the chest, the deltoid muscles in the shoulder and the triceps muscles in the rear of the arm. As well as this, the abdominal muscles will also be affected as they tense to support the body whilst in that bridge like position. One exercise but with multiple benefits.
It should be noted though that with compound exercise such as the Press Up, the Triceps being a relatively small muscle compared with the large Pectoral muscles will tire first, thus leaving the Pectoral muscles not fully utilised.

This can be overcome by doing some isolation exercises just for the pectorals. However, overall I wouldn't worry too much about this as the whole body has the ability to adapt and compensate where necessary.

Isolation exercises.

These are exercises that isolate primarily just one muscle group. For example, concentration curls will primarily just work the biceps. Leg curls will primarily just work just the bicep femoris muscle at the back of the thigh.

Whilst I'm not opposed to isolation exercises, they can be beneficial particularly if you are a professional fitness model or bodybuilder looking to perfect your physique maybe just prior to a contest or photo shoot. Compound exercises however, I feel save time and have multiple benefits. Again, as I keep on emphasising it's your body and therefore your choice.

Not a question that is often spoken, but why ……………

You don't see a Sumo Wrestler with a six-pack.

Now that I've written that chapter title, someone I'm sure will prove me wrong and send me a picture of a Sumo Wrestler with a six pack!
What I am saying here is that you can't exercise one area of your body and expect to lose weight in that area only. So, even if our sumo friend was to do a thousand sit-ups a day, he still wouldn't receive those washboard abs. He may be more muscular on the inside in the abs area, but they would be hidden under pounds of flab. In other words, you can't exercise for spot fat reduction.

Be honest have you ever seen a well-toned male or female with say very flabby thighs or arms? I think not. Generally speaking, they are slim all over or carry excess weight all over.
The body tends to even it all out.

Admittedly we are all built a little differently to each other. Men with excess weight generally get big bellies and with ladies it's generally the tums, bums, and thighs.
Ladies in particular are often saying when it comes to their body, "Oh look at the size of my thighs," Or, "Just look at my hips and my bum." They go on to say what exercises they are doing for that part of the body primarily to remove fat from that area. They then proceed to do a few light isolated exercises for that body part and wonder why the fat is still there!

Yes, they are doing some good in maybe toning up that area, and yes, they may well burn off some fat, but the fat is being removed from the entire body, including the area you want. However, because the result is not what they expected, in the time they expected, they easily give up and go back to eating doughnuts and saying, "Someday," Or, "If only."

When you start to exercise, don't worry if you can't initially see a thinner you in the area of the thighs for example. Fat removal is happening, but you may start to lose the fat in the arms or the back initially more so than in other areas. Be patient and stick at it.

Where's my dumbbells?

The whole point of WOJ is that you don't need any keep fit type of equipment in which to attain that great body. All that equipment will do is add resistance to your muscles so that your body works against that resistance for you to gain muscular development and thus offers you improved shape and tone, help burn fat and reveal you in a better shape than you were a short time ago.

If you want to use your dumbbells or any other piece of exercise equipment, then that's also okay.

Personally, I can feel the movement and tension better in my body by attending my virtual gym or by using bodyweight exercises rather than moving any given external weight.

That's just me.

I'm happy if you want to bin this book and get to a gym and lift those weights. Please, just do something.

Next chapter is exciting as I would like to suggest that you ....

Don't just do a Workout, do a Work In.

You hear it so often in the keep fit circles. "Do you Work out?" This question is often said because someone has noticed how you look or how you may have improved since exercising.

With WOJ of course, you will be, "Working Out," as the phrase goes, but before that you will be doing a "Work In." This simply means that before and whilst doing the exercises you will need to visualise the whole you and how you want to look.

So, for example if you are doing forward squats then you will be concentrating on the buttocks and how you want them to look.

Also, a great boost to your, "Work In," is to talk out loud. Say encouraging things to yourself such as, "I've got great arms and they're growing more muscular each day." Or maybe, "Wow, my stomach is so flat." Or what about, "My shoulders are so shapely."

There is no limit to what you can say, just make sure that it is self-encouraging rather than keep putting yourself down.

Live by faith about how you're going to be in the future and not as you currently are.

Now you may feel a bit daft talking out loud, if so, just talk internally. Your mind and body will react to what you are saying by giving you a more finely honed exercise.

Also, don't get so caught up with numbers. As I've already explained, your mind does not see in numbers, it sees in pictures. It reacts to the demands placed upon it.

If we go back to the dumbbell scenario, the body will react differently to you lifting a 10lb dumbbell to that of a 25lb dumbbell. It will be harder to lift and therefore your body will react differently. Your mind couldn't care less if someone has painted 10lbs or 25lbs on the side of the dumbbells. It's how your body reacts to the lifting that's important.

Likewise, if you are doing press-ups, your body is going to react differently if you do twenty repetitions, rather than 10 repetitions. That's why it can sometimes be so misleading when you follow a workout pattern that someone else has written who doesn't even know you. You then feel a failure because you can't get up to the number of repetitions that they recommend.

Now you may think that I do 50 plus press ups at a time simply bouncing up and down with ease, minutes at a time without breaking into a sweat. If you do, you're wrong. It may surprise you to know that on average I do very few repetitions at a time. Doing press ups in the conventional form, yes, I could do a lot more, but if you want to build a work art, you must be good at your craft and go for every movement with precision and care. No repetition should be wasted.

Think of the Venus De Milo statue. Now I don't know how she lost her arms, but I do know one wrong aggressive move with a hammer can cause more harm than good!

Good form, concentration, slow and purposeful movements are the keys to better reps and therefore better results.

A Sculptor who wants to create a statue in the finest detail wouldn't take a sledgehammer to his stone; if he did, his result would be a pile of rubble. If he wants to create a work of art, then every hit of the hammer on the chisel would be one of precision and care.

A good Sculptor has an instinct; a built-in knowledge and a knowing of just how and where to hit that stone. He already has a picture in mind of what the finished result will look like.

If he doesn't see his masterpiece finished in one week, does he give up and say this is never going to look good?

A good sculptor knows his craft.

He continues chipping away with all the tools and skills that he has until the finished result is achieved. This may take months or even years of work to achieve.

However, the same months have passed irrespective of whether or not he has worked on that statue.

It's the same for you. Time passes anyway. What you do with the time you have been given is up to you.

You can work on improving your knowledge on all the soaps that you watch, such as who is in relationship with who. Or you can gorge on chocolate whilst reading the gossip magazines or you can work on improving you.

You have to build up on that knowing, that inner feeling that you get when you exercise. Getting in tune with your muscles and your body so that you can get the ultimate workout and results. I'm not talking yoga here, or any sort of deep meditation. I'm simply saying feel the effects on your body when exercising to get the maximum benefit from every exercise routine that you perform.
When doing some squats for example, do you feel the burn on the thighs or more so on the hips. With press-ups, is it more on the chest or the triceps, or maybe more on the shoulders?
The more you do it the easier it becomes and the better the results.

One more point regarding the mind before leaving this chapter. When does an ADD become a MINUS?
When A.D.D stands for Attention Deficit Disorder and then has a negative or minus effect on how and who you are.
I am not talking about your attention span here or how much you concentrate on what's going on around you, but rather the amount of attention you receive from others.

Let me explain.
There are a huge amount of people out there suffering from ADD. These people crave attention, affection, applause, and approval. They are always wanting that pat on the back and for people to offer them compliments.
They crave recognition for what they do from the simplest to the mightiest of tasks.
Their lives are one constant, "Look at me, look what I've done, look at how hard I am working compared to others, look what I have achieved. Please notice me, please like me, please accept me, please love me more."

You know what. I get that; its natural, people love the approval of others. In and of itself it's not wrong and it really does makes us feel good.

The problem is the opposite when you do not get the approval you were hoping for. This generally starts from a very early age and the more rejection you got as a child, the more approval you want as you get older.

May I suggest that you be content with who you are right now. You can always build on contentment but be pleased and happy with who you are right now. You're alive and on this earth for a reason. Even if you don't like how you are at the moment, please be content. This is you and this is your starting point to the rest of your life.

When exercising or dieting or whatever you may be doing to improve your life right now, do not do it for the approval of others. This is a big mistake.

Even if you get into your best shape ever and ninety-nine people give you applause, isn't it true that the one person who rejects you or puts you down is the one that will drag you down?

So, what does that have to do with getting that better physical body?
Quite a lot actually.

Get in the best shape for you. For the person in the mirror. Nobody else. That way you are only answerable to you, and it doesn't matter how many negative comments you receive from the naysayers out there. You are responsible for you and nobody else.

Your emotions, your thoughts, your feelings, your confidence. All your responsibility.

You're a God created individual. God loves you and so why not love what He has made. That is YOU. God doesn't create rejects.

When you workout, do it for you. That's not being egotistical but simply sensible. If you do it for others, you are going to get let down. So, get your mind right.

This is important not just for your workout or your body but for your life.

Whether or not you like football; If your team scores, then you can't help but shout ………….

It's a goal and everyone cheers

Everyone should have a goal because as you either reach a goal or score a goal, you can cheer and celebrate.

As you know in any soccer match the game isn't necessarily won by simply scoring one goal. Celebrate yes, but realize that if the opposing team scores one more goal than you. You have lost the match and those previous celebrations will have all been forgotten. You're in it to the end, until the game is over. Then you can truly celebrate.
However, I am not a total killjoy! Going back to a football match for example, isn't it true that if your team wins 6-0 you're still going to cheer every goal?

As well as the end picture in mind you should have mini goals along the way and should celebrate each of these mini milestones. After all you cannot get to a 6-0 win unless you score the 5 goals before it.

Now I know I've said previously that the mind loves to work in pictures and whilst this is true it's also good to have well defined goals such as new measurements or weight targets.
Let's suppose your goal is to reduce your waist size from 40" to 34". I suggest you take a sheet of paper, a private journal, or with today's technology a smart phone or tablet. Write 40" at the top of the page and then work down in ¼" increments 40", 39.3/4", 39.1/2", 39.1/4"…………………34". Each time you reach another ¼" goal, highlight it and celebrate. Go to the movies have a favourite snack, have a glass of wine, simply enjoy the moment. Then work towards the next ¼".

Your mind loves goals. It's like being the captain of a ship. It has to have a destination in mind. It may go a little off track occasionally or go through some rough seas, but the captain always has the final destination in mind.

So, what is your goal? Get it written down. Something visual that you can see and come back to is more powerful than just keeping a number in your head. It makes you accountable to those numbers written down.

Try pinning up a picture of someone you would like to emulate. Maybe a fitness model or actor. Even a friend who managed to get into great shape. Use that picture for inspiration.

Goals come in many forms so find one that you can relate to but break it down into manageable chunks so that your mind doesn't give up from the start.

Feeling tired from all this reading about exercise?

Now is………………..

A time to rest

After doing some Heavy-Duty work on that body of yours, you have to find time to rest. My definition of rest is simply not doing the exercises.
Now I know that a lot of the routines out there will tell you to exercise every day. Well, that's okay if you're just doing some light work such as walking, gentle weight training, swimming etc. However, if you are working hard at these exercises, to the point of virtual failure you are going to have to find time to take more rest.

See it like this. If I was to gently tap your shoulder one hundred times, you would probably find it quite annoying. It may become slightly sore and red and could even be slightly swollen. Recovery however would be fairly rapid. In fact, in just a few hours you may not even feel a thing and the body has returned back to normal.
Now what if I were to strike you very hard on your shoulder, just a few times? In next to no time you would back off and justifiably state how much the shoulder hurts. Examination of the shoulder a few hours later may reveal severe bruising and a throbbing of pain from the shoulder.
Please believe me when I say, I'm certainly NOT into violence. The example above is purely hypothetical.

Now, my questions?
1/   What had the greatest impact on the shoulder?
2/   What hurt the most?
3/   What out of the 2 examples above would take the longest to recover?

Easy questions to answer? Now link those to your workouts. Is your current exercise routine (if you have one), long and boring with plenty of cardio? And if so, are you seeing any great results from all those long hours of working out? Using the first illustration above where someone keeps tapping you on the shoulder you will see that although it became a minor irritation nothing much happened. Why? Because you didn't give your body any reason to change. The only difference was this minor annoyance and inconvenience which your body is well able to cope with. That is why people who do nothing else but go jogging don't have awesome physiques. The long mundane workouts bring the mundane results.

I have never heard anyone say, "Wow, what a physique they must be a marathon runner!"

Now in the second example I emphasised upon the person who hit you hard on the shoulder several times. This led to soreness and bruising and of course a much longer recovery time. However, this happened after just a few hard hits. The whole thing was over and done with in just a few seconds. Likewise, with the exercises, you must give the body a strong enough reason to change and working out hard will do that.

If the body could speak it would say something like, "Wow, this is hard work, I'm not used to this, we're going to have to make some changes here if this happens again. We had better grow the muscles stronger ready for the next workout and if the next workout doesn't come, we can just go back to how we were."

Makes sense? It's a little like going on holiday to same place over and over again. You may like the location but the surprise element is no longer there. It doesn't impact you as much as it did before.

Continually surprise your body by giving it something that it doesn't expect. Work it harder. Increase your intensity level. Change the angle of your body slightly. Add some extra sets and reps. Maybe slow down the rate at which you do the exercise to make it harder.

Remember your body does not want to change. It will resist you all the way. Unless of course you want extra fat! Then generally speaking it is only too happy to oblige.

Increased muscularity on the other hand is no longer a must for survival so your body will resist it.

Long gone of the days when the men had to go off for many days to kill a woolly mammoth in order to give a meaty meal for the family and tribe.

In today's general, sedate society there is no need to carry around any extra muscle because the body doesn't need it to survive.

The only fighting that happens in today's soft society is fighting over the remote control for the TV.

So, unless you have great muscular genetics, you're going to have to go against what your body is telling you to do in order to grow. You must give your body a reason to exercise.
Working out hard, watching your diet, getting plenty of rest, and visualising how you want to look are the fundamentals for this to happen and only you can make this happen.

Do you like precious stones? Well here is ……………

A gem of Information.

It takes energy to keep that fat on your body.
In general terms, every pound of fat that you have on your body burns
approximately 2 calories per day. So, let's say you have 50 lbs of fat on your
body. You are burning that fat irrespective of whether you're reading a book,
watching T.V or driving etc. This equates to approximately, 100 calories per day
even through sedentary activities. In a year this equates to 36,500 calories.
Now as there are around 3,500 calories in 1 pound of fat, your current fat
levels will burn off approximately 10 lbs in a year just through being idle. Good
news you say. I'll eat more so that I'll lose more.
That would be pretty dumb as all you're doing is trying to maintain the status
quo. Staying the same should not be your destination.

Now read this.

For every 1-pound of muscle you have on your body, you are burning
approximately 35 calories per day. As described above this is happening also
through your normal everyday activities.
It takes energy to hold on to your current muscle mass!
So, let's say you're a strong person and have attained through exercise 20 lbs
of additional muscle. This equates to 225,500 calories per year or the burning
up of 73 lbs of fat (a little over 5 stone!).
Sounds too good to be true. Read what an average professional bodybuilder
eats in a day when not training specifically for a contest. They may eat upwards
of 5,000 calories per day and still look good. This is because the muscle on
their body is burning up so many calories.

Now I, and I assume you, are not training to be a Mr. Universe. However, we
can still use this little-known secret for increased fat reduction, and higher
muscle tone that offers a more pleasing look to the body.
As you build the muscle you increase your metabolism and therefore the
ability to burn off greater amounts of fat.

Sure, there may be pills and potions that can also aid fat reduction, but do you really want to take the risks of some of the side effects related to some of these products? Not to mention the expense of some of these products.

The more natural you can be. The better off you are.
Yes, of course a sensible diet is important when trying to achieve the body you want, but don't worry too much.
Let the body do, what the body does best in a natural way.

You work in, you workout, you rest, you eat sensibly, you drink, you get that better body. Simple!

What is often heard in the world of fitness, physique, body shape and exercise is ....

Muscle versus fat

I used to hear it so often. Someone would come along with a great physique and a jealous person would naturally say. "He or she looks good now, but when they're older all that muscle will turn into fat!"

Let's forget the nonsense that muscle turns into fat and fat turns into muscle. Muscle and fat are completely two different things. Yes, both muscle and fat can increase and decrease but they are NOT the same. So, on a body you cannot simply say weight is weight. It's what the weight is made up of that is important.

It's obvious that a 12 stone person with high muscle mass is going to look different to a person that carries a lot of body fat at the same weight.

It's also true that not all bodies are created equal.
Just look at a Heavy Weightlifter compared to a marathon runner. It's pretty obvious that they are poles apart when it comes to the look of the body. Both carry some muscle and some fat. The difference in the proportions to both are quite obvious.

I now want you think in terms of muscular increase and fat decrease and doing the correct exercises and following a sensible diet which are the main factors when it comes to achieving this.

In the old days when purchasing a car, you could have a basic model and it came in one colour, black.
Now you can purchase a car in virtually any colour, with a variety of different types of wheels, upholstery, and a huge number of optional extras. In other words, you can personalise the car to suit you. Have it built your way so that you are pleased with the finished model.
It may cost more than a basic model, but you are not a basic model, are you?

Maybe as you look at yourself in the mirror, you say, well I look like Mr or Mrs average out there. I look like your basic model, nothing special about me. That fine that's just your starting point today.
Please know however that you are the top of the range and when it comes to improvement in your physique.
Dedication to WOJ, bodyweight exercises and sensible eating are the keys to your free upgrade.

I believe that God created you and I to be unique. That means you're special and your standard equipment comes with, "CHOICES."

Fat is far easier to store on your body, but it's difficult to control a wobble. Muscles can be flexed and controlled and shaped and defined. You have control over your body rather than allowing it to control you.

Next time you look in the mirror and don't like what you see, be honest and ask yourself this question. "Is it the excess fat on your body calling the shots? Is it controlling you? Is it leading you down that road of depression?
If it is, then that shouldn't be happening. It's wrong. YOU must control it.

Remember: **You're not random. You're unique and you're defined.**

What follows next is a warning ....

Danger of Diet only.

I know people here, there, and everywhere who are dieting; so, what's the problem? The problem is diet without some form of weight or muscular resistance (body weight or WOJ resistance is okay) exercise.

Dieting is usually associated with eating less and/or eating differently to reduce weight. That part is okay. However, have you ever heard someone say that after their diet they returned to a normal eating habit only to find that their weight had increased above their weight before the diet?

A major UK news organisation said back in 2004 and will remain true forevermore is this.

"Many of the people in the UK put on more weight than they lose when they go on a diet, researchers have found."

A third of people surveyed said they ended up HEAVIER than their original weight only weeks after dieting.

A fifth of those who said they put their weight back on admitted to gaining more than a stone.

A quarter said they got fed up and bored with dieting and nearly half said they found it so hard that they ended up giving in to temptation.

Two thirds put ALL of the weight back on again – nearly half taking only a month to pile on the pounds.

Women were less successful in their quest than the men. Nearly 40% of women ended up being heavier than when they started dieting compared with 20% of men.

It was concluded that, "Fad diets don't work."

So why doesn't this dieting thing work? Simple. As people lose weight through eating less, they not only lost fat but also a degree of muscle. Now as mentioned previously they have just eliminated a portion of their fat burning mechanism called muscle.

Let's look at the following example: -
A person loses say 20 lbs after a dieting only session. However, those 20 lbs may be made up of 15lbs of fat and 5lbs of muscle. "So what." You may say, "Weight is weight; so long it comes off, who cares?" You should care because over the fullness of time this is what occurs. That 5lbs of muscle loss, using the above formula equates to 175 calories less burnt off per day. In a year this equates to 63,875 calories. This then equates to 18lbs of LESS fat removed from the body.
The figures are subject to a lot of variables I know, but they do highlight the problems of diet only without some form of weight resistance type exercise.

Coupled with the above is a hormone in the brain called Leptin. Leptin controls appetite by sending signals to the brain to stop eating. Ever wondered why you feel full after eating; now you know.
It also helps regulate how much energy your body burns throughout the day. Leptin is vitally important in terms of weight loss. It is the safeguard of the body. It stops the body from losing too much weight and will switch off the weight loss when the leptin level drops. Thus, stopping you from dying of starvation.
When your food intake drops so does the efficiency of the Leptin hormone. For it to function properly it needs to have a regular supply of food. The more efficient the Leptin level the more efficient the weight loss.

Science lesson over. How do you think your body would look if you lost 5 lbs of fat but gained 5 lbs of muscle?
Sure, your weight would be the same, but you would certainly look different. Again, this highlights the fact that the mirror is more important than the scales!

Now, what is also common is dieting with added aerobic exercise such as running, swimming, racket sports etc. Again, this is better than nothing as aerobic exercises are great fat burners, and they can add a little muscle tone. Not only that, but when done in moderation is great for overall health.

Please note that aerobic type exercises will indeed burn fat, but only whilst you are doing the exercise. That means that you have to run a lot of miles to burn off just a few calories.

Please don't think I'm knocking all the runners out there. If you want to run, then run. Please realise though if you go for a spot of running and you burn say 250 calories. The next 250 calories you eat will be used to restore your body calorie deficiency.

Also, the plateaus will come. No matter how far you run the fat will stick. It's the body's self- protection mechanism. It needs fat to use as energy, but the body will also keep hold of the fat because it needs it as energy. Makes sense?

I recently heard of one gentleman who was a marathon runner. He ran eighteen marathons, one a year over eighteen years and gained one pound of weight after each one.

As he was now eighteen pounds overweight, he stopped running marathons!

Resistance type training however, providing you work out hard enough will continue to burn calories for around 2 days after training whilst your body recovers from the gruelling workout. Training at the core level means the body has to react to the demands that you put on it.

Think about it; if you do a two-mile run, and you say, "I am absolutely shattered," well you're not really because you could still probably run a little further if you had to. Resistance training however will enable you to reach a point of momentary muscular exhaustion. That's the point when you just simply can't do another press up, or you can't raise yourself in the squat position because your legs are so tired.

That's when changes take place.

I'm not saying that every workout must be like that. Indeed, you should work up gradually to higher and higher levels of resistance and intensity. Also, every now and then you should back off and just do some light movements to help aid recovery. There's only so much the body can take!
Listen to your body. It's vitally important that if you need to rest, then please rest. Take a week of if necessary to allow for full recovery.

Going back to that marathon runner. A good professional runner will complete the race in probably less than two and a half hours. Yes, they're exhausted, however, they could probably run at least another few hundred yards if they had to.
Using the WOJ method you can exhaust the muscles in probably around two minutes, probably even less than that particularly to begin with instead of two and half hours of running time. Also, the fat burning continues in your body well after the exercise period is completed.
To repeat - Am I saying don't jog? No, if you enjoy running then run. Just be open to new ideas and different ways of ridding yourself of unwanted fat other than just aerobic type exercise.

Yes, a good balanced diet is great and should be adhered to, but please add to it a good exercise program on a regular basis.

Do you fancy a change from the traditional way of losing weight?
If it's a yes then it is time to………………………..

Die to diet.

I don't know hold old you are, but whether you are in your teens or well on in years you will have already developed many habits, including a regular eating habit. That is why going on a sudden food deficit such as a crash diet is not going to work very well because you are not internally wired to suit this. You mind is going to rebel because it wants its regular food intake.
Don't get me wrong, if you have a strong will and determination and can stick to it, the weight will come off. Also, if you are very obese it is possible to lose weight more quickly. Please be careful however as you may have problems with nutritional deficiencies, and health issues such as gallstones and with certain individuals, loose skin. Another reason why it is important to discuss a diet and exercise program with your doctor before you begin.
Far better is just a marginal reduction in food and change of food types so that your mind sees and feels very little difference.

I once read a report which observed prisoners in World War II. The ones that had the more serious health problems were those who were overweight when captured. They went from a state of probably overeating to virtually having no food overnight.
As their bodies couldn't cope very well to this new regime it sent the body into a state of shock which in turn caused serious internal health problems.
Sorry to use this sad scenario, but if you are reading this and a serious loss of weight is required then once again get medical advice and lose the weight gradually.
Set up a yearly plan rather than a monthly plan to get yourself back into great shape.

Let's try and get back to some happier reading!
I don't know about you, but I don't like being told I have to eat certain foods of certain types and stick to a maximum number of calories per day.
Eating should be a liberating and pleasurable experience and not a form of bondage to certain foods only.

Salads are okay but not all the time, please! Same goes for, "greens." Yes, I know they are healthy and of course I eat fruit and vegetables, but I also enjoy the odd pizza, or chocolate, or cake, or crisps, or chips and so the list goes on. If I had to put a ratio on good food to, "junk," type food I would say do 75-80% good and the other I would leave to your discretion.

"I'm so overweight," you say, and now you're telling me I can eat anything? No, I'm not saying that. I'm simply saying that you must make your own decisions based upon what you want your destination to be. If you want to lose weight then eat less of the so-called bad foods, eat healthier meals, add weight resistance exercises, and do some aerobics as well if you want to.

So often you hear or read about so called experts telling you what you should and shouldn't eat. They tell you if you eat this or that you will look like him or her.
Just look at the people on the advertisements, particularly around the Summer and the beach season. Will you really look like the ladies with the hourglass figure if you eat their brand of cereal? I doubt it!
Every person is different and there are so many variables involved, because no two body types are the same.

If you're serious about reaching your destination, then YOU HAVE TO TAKE RESPONSIBILITY FOR YOURSELF. It's not my job to look after you, it's your job.

I know it's natural to take the path of least resistance, and that's why we're so quick to blame someone else when things don't work out for us.
This equipment is no good. I don't lose weight by going to that gym. I gained weight when I ate that supermarket's carrots and I not going to shop there anymore. Sounds daft I know, but you'll be amazed at how many people have to administer blame to someone or something for their own lack of effort.

I'll say it again, "YOU TAKE RESPONSIBILITY FOR YOU." That way you will get out of life what YOU put into it.
The only person to blame for anything in this life is you.

Habit, habit, habit on the right words, the right thoughts, the right actions until they become natural.

Now back to diet basics. I know I mentioned above about sticking to a 75-80% healthy diet, but that doesn't mean you absolutely have to eat five chocolate bars per day to make up the other 20-25%. That would be silly. Unless of course you want to do a commercial for, "Zits are me."
What I do is simply try to be sensible and enjoy a varied diet with a good variety of all food types. The emphasis should be more on carbohydrates and proteins and a little less on fatty or high sugar items, but I will leave your precise choices up to you.

A gentleman once told me how he lost six stone in weight over the course of a few years and without really trying. Also, to the best of my knowledge he didn't even do any additional exercises.
Of course, you want to know how? He simply served his meals on a medium size dessert plate rather than a normal size dinner plate. Thus, his meals were approximately 10 to 20% smaller. Simply put, your mind is tricked in to thinking it is still eating a full plate of food.
This is of course true, but there is just less of it.

Eat less, weigh less.
Add exercise and weigh less, faster.

Also, forget the guilt trip. I've seen people who get so uptight if they've eaten five extra calories that day or have given into temptation and eaten an extra slice of cake. Life is there to be enjoyed, so don't sweat the small stuff.

Think about it; if food wasn't meant to be a pleasure, then you wouldn't require a tongue with so many built in taste buds would you? We're made this way for a reason.
I know this isn't exact science and deep dietary exploration; but it's not meant to be. I have a philosophy of keeping things fun and simple.
If food is a big thing for you then by all means go and get books on the subject. Study calories and food breakdown if you want to; it is just not for me.

If you're overweight as so many people are, then start with at least reducing meal sizes just marginally. Maybe have a jacket potato instead of chips. Add extra salad. Change a desert from ice cream to fruit.

Why not save that chocolate bar and use it as a reward? Maybe when you can do 5 press ups in good form. Or maybe 10 squats.
What about that goal you have of walking a mile? Keep it simple and pleasurable.
As I mentioned in a previous chapter, set yourselves small goals, reach them and move on to the next.

Please, don't get yourself stressed about the whole diet thing. Life is too short for that. Keep it simple and enjoy yourself.

That's easy for you to say…………………………

But my mind keeps telling me to eat the stuff, I know I shouldn't eat.

So called non-healthy foods can be taken, but just in moderation. Maybe eat snacks as a treat for maybe just 2 days a week. Look forward to those days when you can say, "It's snack day," and go and eat a chocolate bar or a cake. Maybe use it as a reward when you reach a specific fitness or weight loss goal when creating the new you, as I mentioned previously.
If you really do have an addiction to maybe one or more types on unhealthy food, the following tactics may help.

Let's use chocolate as an example.

1. You can go and eat a box of chocolates and then feel sick and guilty at the same time.
   Not recommended.

2. You can eat one chocolate and say, "That's it for today. I'll have another one tomorrow."
   Better.
   However, once you start it's difficult to stop. One chocolate leads to another, then another until the box is gone and you say, "Well how did that happen?"

3. You can shout out at the top of your voice, "I JUST QUIT CHOCOLATE." Better still. Easier if there is no one else around. However, this method will jolt the body into reacting. Particularly if you do it often enough and add emotion to it as you shout it out.

4. You can however take things to a much deeper and effective level. Try this: -

   Visualize yourself eating chocolate and then have an utter dislike for it. See yourself heaving at the thought of having to eat it.

That brown stuff in your mouth is causing you to want to spit it out as quickly as possible. See yourself running to the bathroom and spitting it out. Suddenly the taste is so awful you can't even stand the sight of it. The worst you make the picture in your mind the easier it will be to resist it.

Make the colours bright and the sounds loud. Actually move your mouth round and round in an eating motion. Make it a very real experience. Each time the thought of chocolate comes to you think of it as a minus 10 on your scale of 1 to 10 on your food list.

Repeat this thought pattern often. Especially if that bar of creamy milk chocolate is calling your name and within a very short time your love of chocolate will be greatly diminished.

I'll say it again, be sensible. Don't be in bondage to totally healthy foods. In fact, so called healthy food are not always as healthy as you may think. For example, low fat foods sometimes mean high sugar foods, which aids the body in storing fat. Far better is to fill up on natural fruit and vegetables. Some meat (unless you're a vegetarian) and dairy foods are also good but watch out for too much fat and as I said, enjoy an occasional treat.

Did you know that "Nature arbours a vacuum?" What does that mean?
In scientific terms it means that if you have an empty space you want to fill that space with something.
A little like in your home. If you have a big blank wall, you will most likely put a picture or a mirror on that wall to fill the space.
So, for example if you try and rid your thoughts, emotions, and feelings for say fizzy type drinks, which as you know contain a lot of sugar and therefore can add unwanted weight; you have to fill that void with something else. Maybe a cup of tea, a glass of milk, some chilled water.
The important thing here is that you fill that space with something a little healthier than the one you're trying to give up.

Let's move on to a drinking problem……………………………..

Don't Forget to Drink.

Very few people take drinking seriously!

Drinking what? Water of course.
Most people know that they have to drink and therefore assume that all drinks are created equal. As long as I am drinking something, which is better than nothing then I must be okay right? Well not really. If you drank nothing but fizzy drinks it wouldn't be too long before you noticed weight gain in all the wrong places as well as having negative health issues.
Unused sugar levels must go somewhere and do something. Some stored fat is good as you need this to live, but excessive amounts? Well you know the result of that.

Let's talk water.
On average the human body is made up of around 50-65% water. However, the percentage is not divided equally around the body. The brain for example is around 85% water. That's why when you lack water, one of the first things to happen is that you can't think properly, and you lose some mental clarity.
The muscles are just over 70% water. Again, don't drink enough and fatigue and tiredness sets in.
It's interesting to know that your body fat contains only around 15% water.
Some people think that the more I sweat when working out, the more weight I must be losing. In reality it's making virtually no difference.
Sure, you're burning calories, which in turn equates to weight loss but the fluid you lose through your sweat glands is very minimal.

Water is essential to life. It helps keep skin supple. It helps keeps your body at the right temperature, hence your doctor tells you to keep taking fluids when you're suffering from colds, flu etc.
Water gets rid of the body's natural waste through urine. It offers lubrication to the joints and make digestion of food possible.

At the end of a hard day have you ever felt that your back aches, you have a headache, your eyes hurt, and you feel totally fatigued?

One reason is that you have probably told yourself umpteen times during the day how tired you feel and therefore your body is acting on your instructions on how to feel lousy.
The other reason may well be that you have not drunk enough water. Stop, listen to your body, act on what you feel and if you need to drink, then drink. IT'S ESSENTIAL TO HEALTHY LIVING.

I would recommend that you get into the habit of always having with you a water bottle. Keep a few small bottles topped up in the refrigerator. As you drink, top up.
You probably already know that there are zero calories in water.
However, what you may not know is that it takes energy and therefore calorie-burn to heat up the water that you drink to body temperature. Not only is cold water more refreshing but it has the added benefit of weight loss as well as the scores of health benefits.

How much water is good for me?
Well a common answer you may have heard is 6-8 glasses a day. This is a bit vague as it depends upon the size of the glass you are drinking from.
You may want to discover what is best and practical for yourself. Personally I try and drink up to 3 to 4 pints a day. This may sound excessive, but I have not had any health defects from this amount of water and it has helped reduce my waist line.

My suggestion is that you try and increase your cold-water intake in small increments and note the changes in your general wellbeing.

Now for some very fancy words that describe how you are made up.

So ....

What about body types. Am I or are you primarily Ecto, Endo, or Meso?

Well firstly the above names are abbreviations for ectomorph, endomorph, and mesomorph. These are simply different body types, and everyone is a mixture of all three types. It's just that a lot of us lean more towards one or maybe two of these types.
Let me explain.

Ectomorphs are built like a stick. You know those annoying types who can eat a mountain of food and never put on an ounce. They are usually thin in appearance, have narrow wrists and ankles and usually quite small heads. These types make very good long-distance runners. They always seem to be on the go because they have bundles of energy.
These people have a high metabolism and don't generally find burning off food a problem. They will also probably maintain a set weight for years and years and may only start to put on weight as they reach middle age and beyond.

Endomorphs are those people who only have to look at a pea and put on a pound. They often have roundish chubby faces. Mainly because of the weight they have put on.
They generally have a slow metabolism meaning that it takes longer for their bodies to burn up excess calories.
The problem for the people with this body type is that because of their easy weight gain they often find it more difficult to exercise. They may also suffer from sore joints and other medical ailments due to the effect of excess weight. As exercising may be difficult for them, they may downward spiral by doing less and less whilst gaining more and more weight. Leading to an increase in health problems and often mental concerns such as depression.

Mesomorphs are a men's dream. This body type is the natural muscular type. I heard of a man who won a bodybuilding contest without ever lifting a weight just because he was naturally muscular.
As this type has a lot of natural built in developed muscle, they also find it fairly simple to maintain a reasonable weight because calories just seem to burn off

them. Well at least prior to middle age, and then this type seems to pile on the pounds without any additional exercise.

I know of a lady who falls well into this category. She is approximately 5' 6" tall, weighs around fifteen stone. However, she looks like she weighs around thirteen stone. This is because the weight she carries is mainly muscle. Muscle is denser than fat. So 1lb of muscle on her body takes up far less room that 1lb of fat. Hence, she is heavy but doesn't have the size of some who is predominantly endomorphic weighing fifteen stone.

Now, as I explained earlier, no one is 100% ecto, endo or meso. We are made up of all three types but may swing more towards one type than another.

There are also lots of other variables and it's worth noting that body types can change throughout a person's life due to lifestyle, age, hormones, genes, stress, food patterns, to name but a few.

Please don't caught up too much with analysing yourself to a finite degree.

I only wanted to point out these facts to make you aware that we are all different.

Please, please, please realise that you may never have the body of your idol, and neither should you because simply put you should not have any idols. I will say it again, being inspired by people is fine. They can help towards how you want to look and that's great.

Why place someone else on a pedestal when they are just as important as you are? Admire people yes, but please remember they are unique in the way they look and both you and I are unique in the way we are.

You were created special, and you should love yourself regardless of what you currently look like.

Your body changes throughout your lifetime, hopefully for the better through the exercises you will read about later.

So hopefully by now I have covered most of the basics you need to know to get you from where you are now to where you want to be.

Enjoy relationships? Good, because now is the time for…………

Choosing the Right Partner

By partner, I'm talking about training partner. Not a must. In fact, when I exercise, I do it alone. That's just me. However, if you do want to exercise with someone and many people do, then that's great.
That's another reason why gyms and fitness centres are so popular. As well as great places to exercise they also have a strong social aspect to them. It is good to train with someone.

Without even reading any further, you already probably know who you can ask and who you can't. Don't just pick someone because there your best friend. Find that person who is as keen as you are to get into great shape. Remember that whoever you choose, they too should be in it for the long haul.

Your training partner should be there to inspire and encourage you. To urge you on to do one more rep, take you beyond your own pre-set boundaries. Likewise, you should do the same for them. Even a little healthy competition is good.

Please also ensure that your training buddy isn't the sort of person that is a nonstop chatterbox, who just loves to talk about everything from football to soap operas to politics. The talking can come later.
Whilst exercising the only chat should be about the task in hand such as encouraging and motivating that person on to give it their best.

As well as exercising with them, also make sure that you are well able to motivate yourself to train without them. After all, if your friend goes on holiday for 2 weeks are you going to take a fortnight break from training?

There is a saying that any one person is the average of the five people he or she hangs around with. This goes for the way you think, your opinions, your words, your finances etc. Without realising it, those close people that you hang out with, are having a major effect on your life and are influencing you more than you realise.
Surround yourself with happy and joyful friends that can be great encouragers.

Please have fun during your exercise times. It makes the whole experience far more enjoyable.

Please pick your friends wisely and why not get a WOJ group going?

What follows next is a really difficult question. Particularly for you ladies........................

What Shall I Wear?

Such an important question! To some people this is the most important thing in the whole of their exercising life. Why? Because instead of thinking of their workout they think about what other people may be thinking about them whilst they're working out.

Remember what I said at the start of this book, people are like sheep, and they all want to blend into the flock. Therefore, they want to wear what they feel others may think appropriate.
Free range chickens run around the hen coup clucking away all day long. Eagles on the other hand soar high, high above the chickens and are the masters in their space.
Are you the chicken or the eagle? Your choice.

In reality, it doesn't really matter what you wear. Believe me when I say that it's not important if your t-shirt doesn't match your jogging trousers. So long as you can move about and have free movement, you can wear a suit and tie or baggy jumper and jeans. It really doesn't matter. Just be comfortable.

However, please leave the stilettoes in the wardrobe. Focus on what you are doing rather than looking at that person over there with the latest style of sweatshirt!

You're working on what's under the clothes. So, don't focus on what you think other people are thinking about because they too are probably thinking more about themselves than you. Focus on what you need to be focused on and that is the exercises ahead and the effect they will have on your body.

You need to get in the right frame of mind as you are about to give all your attention to each repetition. Each small blow of the hammer from the sculptor is like each movement you make as you rep back and forth. The hammer and chisel represent the exercise and YOU are the finished work of art!

So here they are: **The Exercises.**

The first section is the **WOJ** exercises that give you totally flexibility. Exercises that can literally be done at any place, anywhere, any time.
Followed by **Body Weight Exercises.**

A few reps can literally be done in seconds. As you get into the habit of WOJ exercises you will find that you will be doing them without even thinking about it.

So now is the time to switch planets, for you are about to commence..............

Walking on Jupiter (WOJ)

So, why walk on Jupiter? As mentioned in the Introduction, walking on Jupiter, if it were physically possible would be incredibly difficult due to the strong gravitational pull. However, if you lived on the planet then your body would have to adapt. It would therefore have to get naturally stronger as it adapted to the planet's super gravitational pull.

This means that your arms would increase in strength by simply lifting them. Shoulders would get broader and wider by lifting your arms above your head. Legs, more powerful and shapely by simply going from crouch position to standing.

As your muscular development increases so will your fat burning mechanism also increase.

The exercises that follow use that same philosophy. If we can copy the movements that you might use in the gym such as Bench Press, Pull Downs on the Lat machine or Bicep Curls then we're getting close to where we need to be. What if we could combine some of those exercises into one movement? The big difference is that we don't need to be at the gym or lift the weights to produce the results we want.

We are going to basically trick the mind into thinking it is lifting the weights by tensing the muscles for each movement as though we were lifting against a resistance.

This is where it also gets very interesting. What if I was to tell you that you can do multiple exercises, working multiple muscles for multiple gains in one movement in a fraction of the time it would take by doing the exercises in the gym?

Is this the perfect system to train anywhere and at any time? No, because there is no perfect system out there. However, in my opinion it comes pretty close!

Some of you may be asking, "How do I monitor progress if there are only imaginary weights? How can I tell if I am upping the poundage that I'm lifting or the number of repetitions?

What do I write in my training log?" Basically, nothing.

Why not simply go by the results that you can see in the mirror, on the scales, or by using the tape measure.

I think it's worth saying again. Your body couldn't care less what the numbers are on the side of the weights. It's the effort, intensity, and downright hard work that your body will react to.

If you keep constant tension on the muscles throughout the range of the exercises, you will simulate that of actually lifting the physical weights.

This is certainly not some wimpy alternative of going to the gym. A few minutes into your routine, you will know what I am talking about.

Believe me, you will tire and tire quickly.

At many gyms you will find people trying to do reps with a weight that is far too heavy for them anyway. Form goes out the window and in comes an injury that can sometimes take months to get over.

Remember again. You are training your body. Not your ego!

Just a word of caution. I know you're enthusiastic and can't wait to get started but as with any exercise routine, warm up a little, slightly tense the arms and relax, repeat this a few times. Do a few squats. Reach to the ceiling, stretch your limbs. Even do a few standing press ups against the wall.

You're basically saying to your body, get ready for what's about to come.

The WOJ Exercises

So, at last we have come to the WOJ and the Body Weight Exercises.

Irrespective of which of the exercise you are doing, please take care to read each execution of the exercise carefully.

Try not to jerk the body through the movement but rather let each movement be a masterclass of execution. Remember you are not simply going through the motions of doing a number of repetitions, 1,2,3,4........10 finished, but rather doing the exercise until you feel that that is enough and I can't do any more. That is the stage where the body changes and results happen.

Remember why you are doing what you are doing. That is tensing the activated muscles and concentration on the movement and the muscles you are using, whilst thinking about the ultimate look that you want.

Here's the list of the basic WOJ exercises. Again, if you want to add your own or deviate the movement slightly from the descriptions below then that's fine. Be flexible. I won't mind!

Upper Body Wonder 1
Whole Arm Movement (WAM)
Shoulder Lat Flap
Upper Body Wonder 2
Pec Push
Breast Stoke
Curlext
Jupiter Lunge

Exercise name: Upper Body Wonder 1
Benefits: Chest, Shoulders, Lats (Wide back muscle), Biceps and Triceps
Mindset: Focus your thoughts on the above muscles that will be utilised. A full broad chest that shows off density and shape rather than a hollow flat appearance. Broad wide shoulders. A wonderful tapered back and shapely arms.
Maybe you have pictures that can emulate the look you want to have for these certain body parts.

I call this exercise the Upper Body Wonder because it stimulates most of the upper body in just one exercise and replaces three exercises that you would normally do in the gym. (Bench press, Forward shoulder Press and Lat Pull Down).

To start this exercise, you can either sit or stand. Put both arms out in front of you at chest height. Now a make a fist with both hands. Draw back the arms so that they are now level with the front of the chest (Picture 1)

Now tense the arms to around 80-90% of your maximum and keep that tension there.

You will automatically find that you are tensing the chest and back muscles at the same time. Feeling this?

Now keeping the tension on the arms, push the arms forward, straight out in front of you (Picture 2)

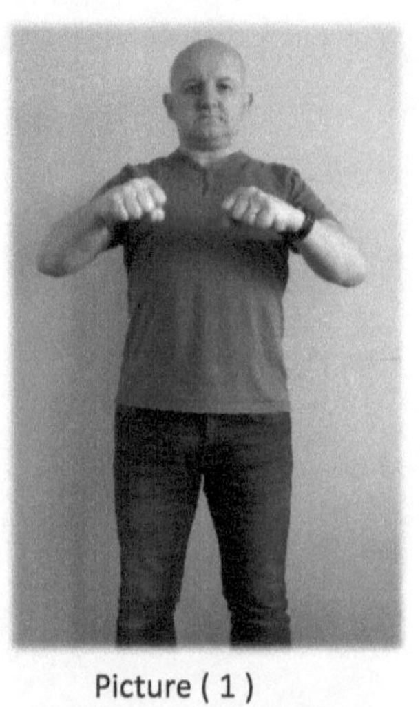

Picture (1)

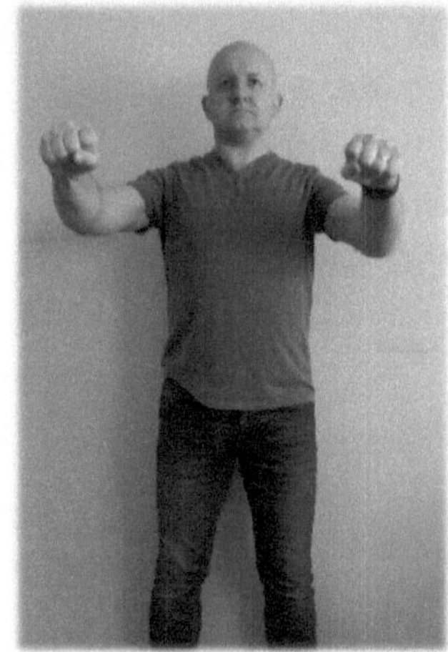

Picture (2)

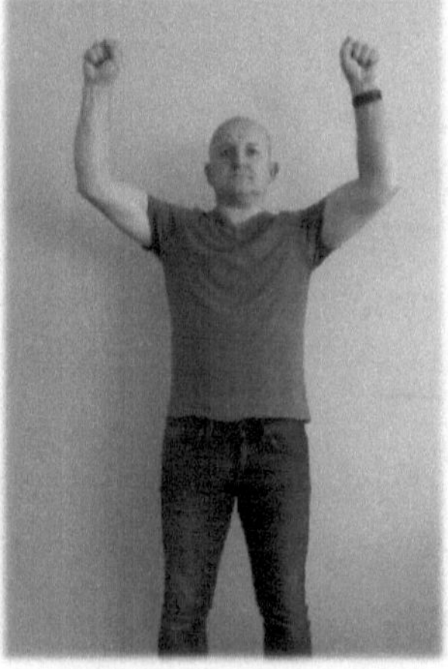

Picture (3)

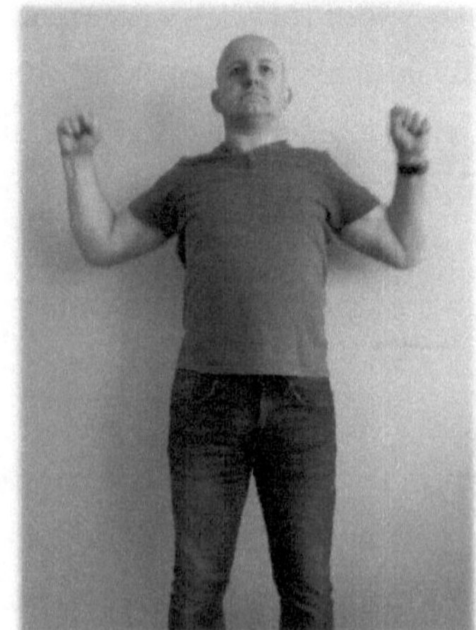

Picture (4)

This simulates the movement of a Bench press exercise, except that you are standing vertical instead of lying on a bench horizontally.

Now once the arms are straight out in front of you (still under tension), raise the arms up so that they finish over the top of your head around shoulder width apart. This part of the exercise will stimulate the shoulder muscles (Picture 3)

Now start to lower the arms NOT back in front of you, but rather in a vertical position, straight down so they are in line with the shoulders (Picture 4). As you do so you will feel the muscles in the side of the back come into play. Your hands should now be line with the sides of your chest.

Remember, keep the muscles tensed all the time throughout the movement. Now push out the arms in front of you once again to repeat the movement.

One repetition should last approximately 8 to 10 seconds.

To begin with you will probably tire fairly quickly after just a few repetitions. That's normal.

Try and build up to 10 – 15 repetitions.

This is a great all-round upper body developer.

By doing this exercise just 2 or 3 times a week you will start to build up strength and before long start to notice differences in your physique.

Exercise name: Whole Arm Movement (WAM)

Benefits: Biceps, Triceps and forearms

Mindset: As this exercise primarily focuses on the arms, I would ask that you visualise the arms of someone you admire such as the Action Hero's you see on today's TV or Cinema. Whether they be male or female, I have to admire the great shape that many of these people get into for their starring roles. You don't have to be the biggest, but great shape and tone even on a small arm can look great.

This WAM exercise replaces the normal Bicep Curl, Tricep Pushdown and Wrist Curl that would normally be done in the gym. Again, three exercises in one movement.

This exercise once again can be done in either a standing or sitting position. If seated, please ensure that you are in a chair with no arms so that free movement can be obtained.

Begin with your arms simply hanging down at your side. Now make a fist with both hands and turn you fists upwards towards you forearms. You will now notice that your entire arm is now tensed (picture 1).
Keeping your elbow and upper arm static, raise your forearm in a 90-degree angle so that your hands are just a few inches away from your shoulder (picture 2). This is very similar movement to a bicep curl. Keep the tension high throughout the movement. You should now be looking at the top half of your fingers.

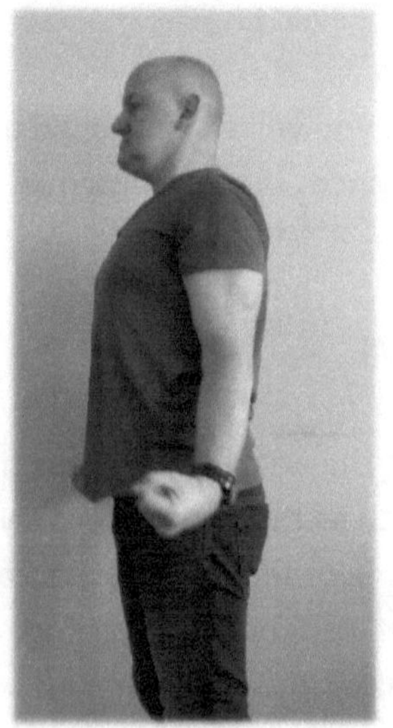

Picture (1)

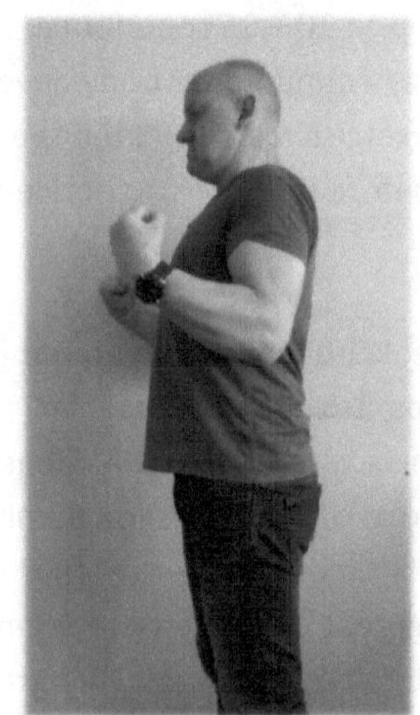

Picture (2)

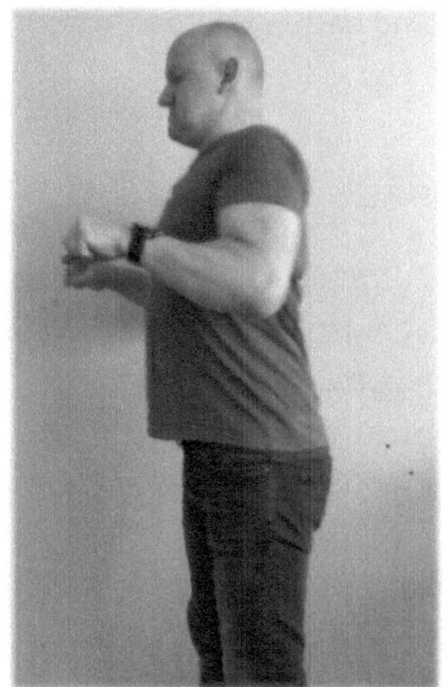 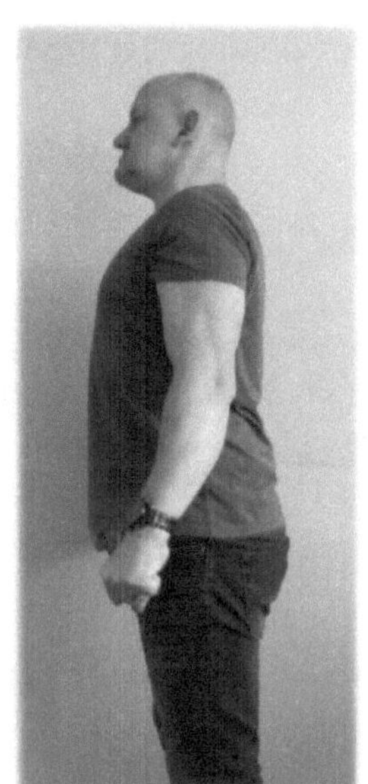

Picture (3)   Picture (4)

Once in that position turn your hands and forearms through 180 degrees so that you are now looking at the backs of your hand (picture 3). This now stimulates the Tricep muscles on the backs of the arm.

Keeping the elbows stationary, lower the arms under tension until they are down by your side (picture 4).

Once back in the starting position turn the hands through 180 degrees so that you are now looking at the front of your hands (picture 1) and repeat the process.

Once again aim for 10-15 repetitions at least 2 or 3 times a week. The greater the tension the more difficult it will be. This has the same effect as adding more weight to a barbell, dumbbell, or exercise machine.

Exercise name: Shoulder Lat Flap

Benefits: Shoulders, sides of the back

Mindset: As in the WAM exercise mentioned above, this exercise primarily works shoulders and back. So once again see yourself with those wide broad shoulders and lean tapered back, leading down to that small defined waistline.

The advantage of working the shoulders and back is that they can be seen from both front and back and give you a great overall look.

This exercise can be completed in either the sitting or standing position.
Start with your hands down by your side. Palms facing inwards (Picture 1).
Make a fist and tense both shoulders and arms. Now start to raise your arms in line with your body so you form a cross type shape. Imagine a bird flapping its wings. That's the sort of movement you require.
DO NOT lock your arms but rather bend them slightly.
At the top position (Picture 2), your arms should be around the level of the top of your head.
The upwards movement works the shoulders. On the return position you will work the sides of the back.
Now as you lower the arms in the same way you raised them, tense the back muscles as well as the arms and keep that tension on until the hands are once again fully lowered.
At the bottom of the movement, your hands should be touching the sides of your hips.

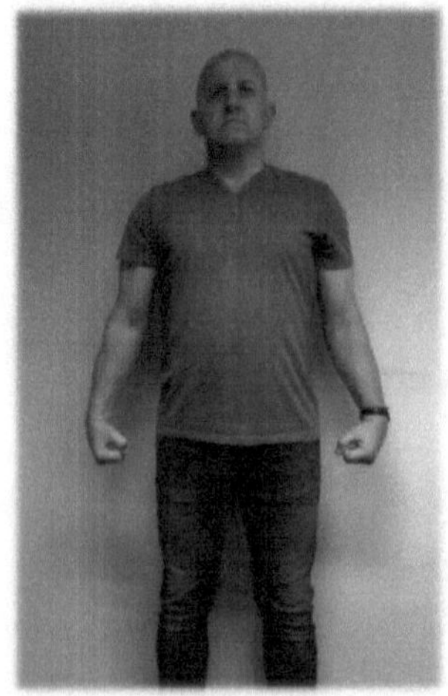

Picture (1)

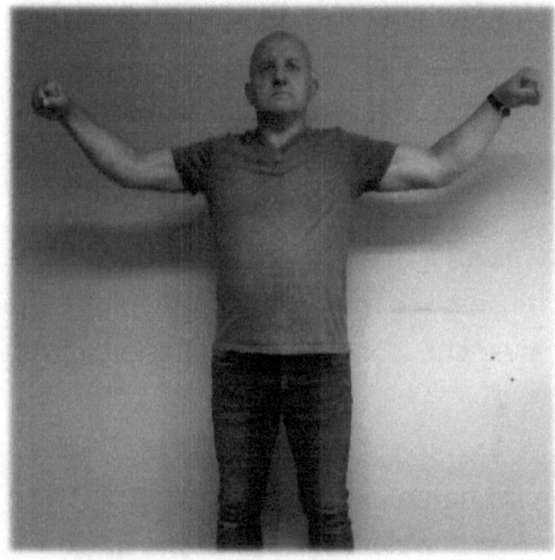

Picture (2)

Each repetition should be done in a slow and deliberate manner and fully concentrate on your muscles being activated. Feel the pump.

Over the coming weeks, you should be able to build up to the customary 10-15 repetitions. Feel free to do 2 or 3 sets, 2 or 3 times a week.

Exercise name: Upper Body Wonder 2
Benefits: Shoulders, Upper back (Trapezius), Chest and Triceps
Mindset: For most people the upper back won't be considered too important. Why? Because it is mainly out of sight, out of mind. You can't see it, unless you have a strange mirror configuration. However, from the front, this area of the back can be seen as it is the muscle that sits between the shoulder and the neck. Over developed and it can give way to a more displeasing look rather than that of a complimentary appearance.
Regarding mindset, I would say once again, view people who have an overall broad shouldered, wide back appearance. The likelihood is, that they have also developed the trapezius muscle, giving the back a more complete look.
This exercise is best done in the standing position.
With arms by your side, ensure that the backs of your hands are facing forward when making that fist and tensing the whole arm.
Remember as you tense, think that you are holding 2 heavy weights down there by your side (Picture 1).

Tip: Never underestimate the power of words. This may be a little strange but speak to your body. If you want bigger and broader shoulders then speak to the shoulders, tell them that they must grow. Tell the chest that it is getting larger with defined pectorals.
Arms, you're getting shapelier, with biceps that can be seen through your shirt.
Ladies, tell that waist that it has to get smaller.
Speak it and visualise it. These are powerful tools that has a great effect on your finished result.

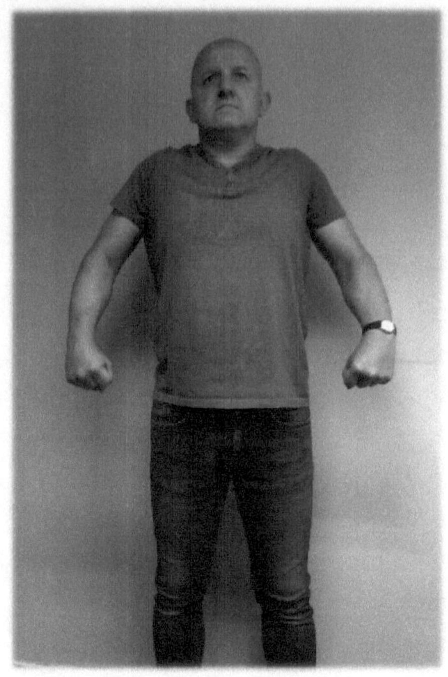

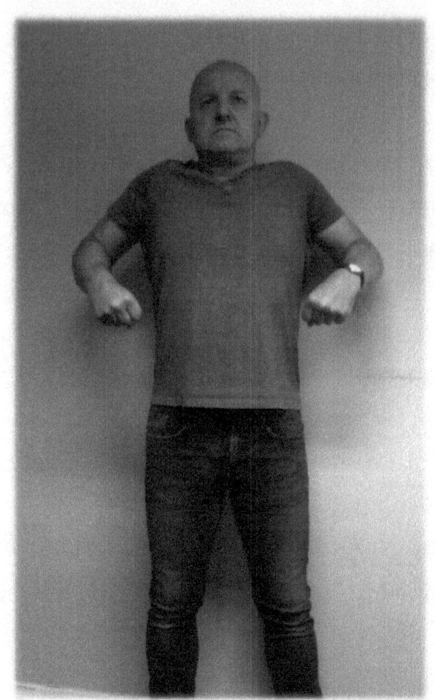

Picture (1)   Picture (2)

Now start to raise and bend the arms simultaneously as well as raising the shoulders. (Think of when you were a bored child and just shrugged your shoulders when asked to do a tiresome task). In the top position your hands should be level with your lower chest and your elbows sticking out from your side. Like a hen flapping its wings.

Now as you lower the arms (still under tension), you should be able to feel and stimulate the pectorals (chest muscles) and the triceps on the backs of the arm.

See what I mean about working multiple muscle groups in one exercise?

The greater the intensity the more quickly you will be fatigued. Greater the fatigue the more the muscles are being stimulated.

Don't be afraid to stop and take a few deep breathes and carry on.

How much is enough? Basically, you will know. You will simply feel shattered and know that enough is enough. Rest and recover.

Exercise name: Pec Push
Benefits: Chest and Biceps
Mindset: Basically put, men look good with well-developed pectorals. It gives that barrel chested look rather than that of an ironing board. You see well developed pecs and you think that guy works out. He looks after his body. He's got energy, power, and strength. His clothes fit better. He walks better, He exudes energy.

Although you cannot see the pecs directly on a lady, due to the bust, the pecs are still there and gives a greater overall look to the body. It increases the ratio of chest to waist and offers an overall improved look.

As for biceps, we all know the look of that peak on an upper arm. Again, it tells us that this person works out.

Very often the arms are the only limbs on show, so again it's important to mould those arms into a well-defined shape showing off both biceps and triceps.

Look for all aspects of, "Good arms," there are plenty are images out there to inspire you.

This exercise can be done seated or standing. Arms should be out from your sides and horizontal with palms facing outwards to make that cross type shape (Picture 1).

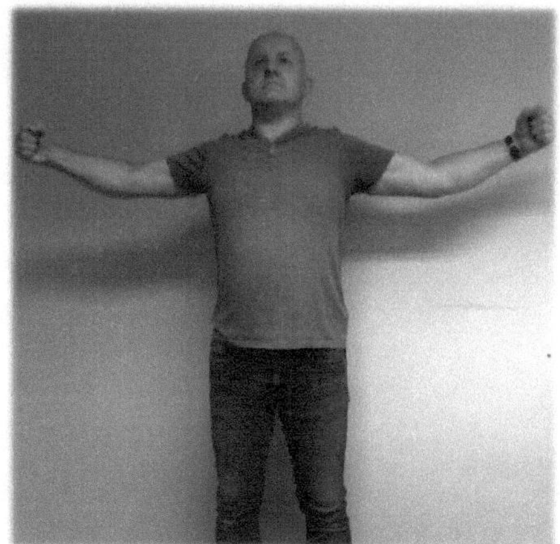

Picture (1)

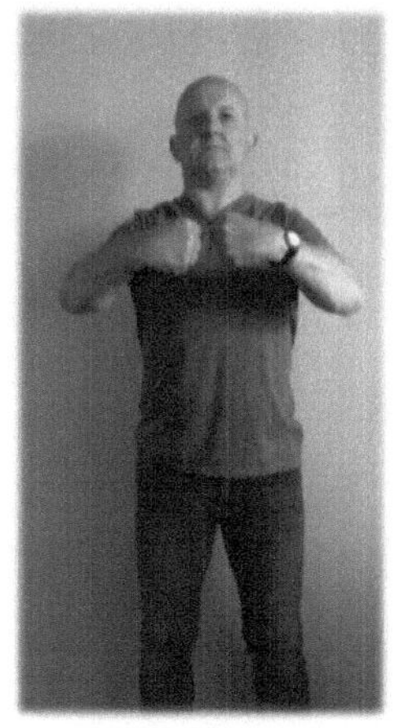

Picture (2)

Make a fist with both hands and tense those arms. Now bring both hands in together in a forward arc so that hands touch, level with your chest (Picture 2). As you do this you should be able to feel the tension on your chest and arms. In the gym this is the exercise you would do on a Pec Dec machine.

As with all exercise in the WOJ section, aim for the 10-15 reps with intensity, at least 2 times a week.

Exercise name: Breaststroke
Benefits: Chest, Shoulders, Back, Arms.
Mindset: A strong and full chest, Wide and broad shoulders, strong muscular back and shapely strong defined arms are all easy to imagine. You'll find all of these attributes on the big screen heroes or on the cover of the fitness magazines. Try any search engine and you've got an infinite array of images you can use for inspiration.
If they can achieve it, then you can achieve it.
The better body is within your reach. Just use your imagination and become inside the person you want to be on the outside.

On to the exercise. Think of the Breaststroke done in swimming and replicate it (without the water of course).
Do this and you can't go far wrong with this exercise.

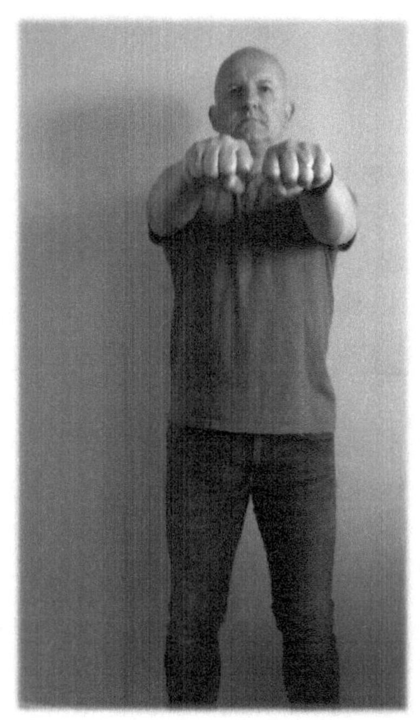

Picture (1)

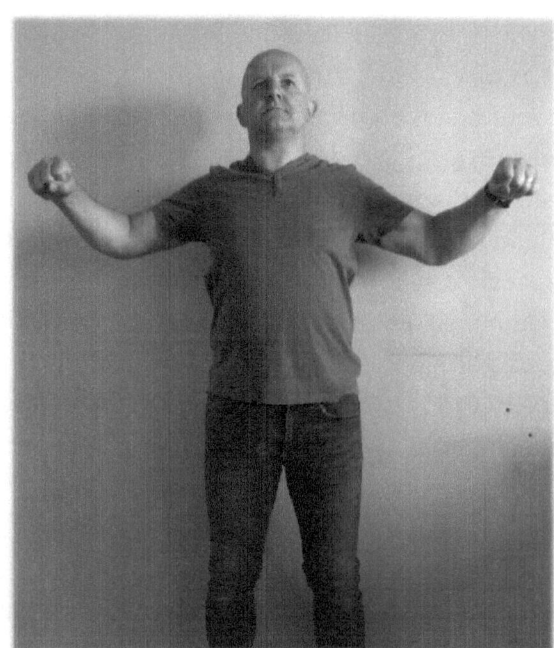

Picture (2)

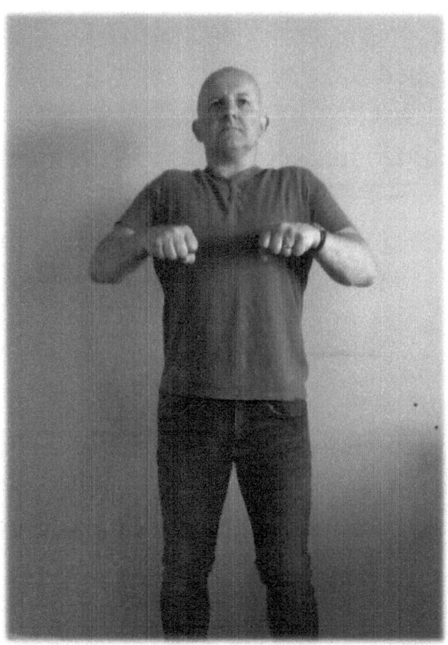

Picture (3)

Standing or sitting again is fine for this exercise.

Start by placing your arms out in front of you at chest height (picture 1), so that your hands are touching each other. Now make a fist with both hands and tense both arms. Now in a large arc swing your arms out so that you form a cross type shape with your body (picture 2). Without stopping (this should be a continuous flow of movement) bring your hands back in front of you so that they meet right in front of your chest (picture 3). Push them forward (remember all under tension) so they are back in the starting position in an extended arm position in front of you (picture 1).

Go for 10 to 15 repetitions. Rest and repeat. This is a hard but great exercise for the upper body. Put every effort into it, to get every bit out of it.

Legs:

Now for the legs. If I'm honest the best exercise ever for the legs is simply the Squat. Depending upon body position you can emphasise the hips, butts, and thighs. This exercise is covered in detail in the Body Weight Exercises section. However, WOJ could be applied to the squat as you can raise the body slowly as though there is a great weight (increased gravity) working against you.

So instead of raising your body quickly, slow it right down as though you are rising up in a slow-motion fashion.

The slower you go, the harder the exercise.

For now, I would like to welcome you to another exercise which involves only raising one leg at a time and thus enables you to concentrate more on the movement.

Exercise name: Leg Curlext

Benefits: Quadriceps (Large muscle on the front of the thighs) & Bicep Femoris (Muscle group at the back of the thigh).

Mindset: Great upper legs. Plain and simple. I'm sure we all know people with legs they admire. It's one of the parts of the body that we all crave over. Particularly you ladies.

I know that guys tend to go for upper body development and often ignore the legs, because 99% of the time they're covered over.

Another reason for the legs getting neglected is that leg work is such hard work. The thighs have large muscle groups and therefore take a lot of work, which requires a lot of oxygen. Training legs is certainly a heavy breathing exercise. The results however, are worth it.

This exercise is best performed by sitting on the edge of a firm chair. Something like a dining or office type chair will be fine.

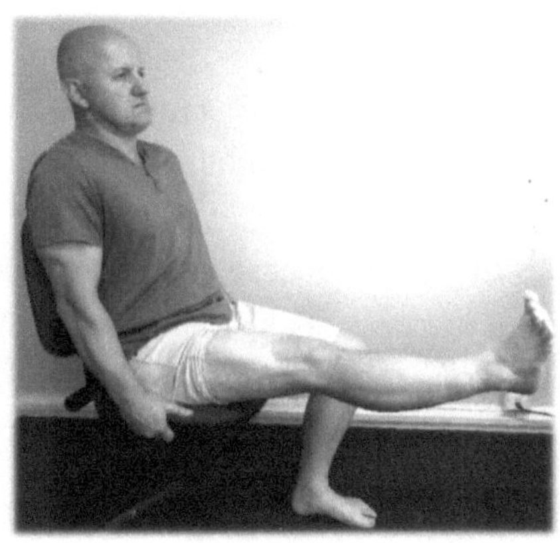

Picture (1)

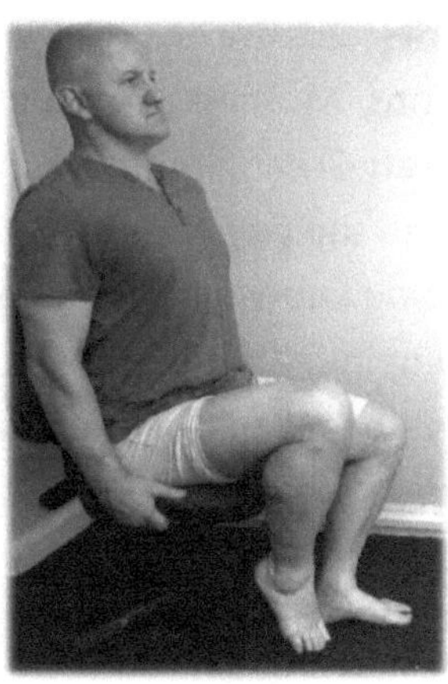

Picture (2)

With one leg resting on the floor for support, stretch out the other leg so that only your heel is resting on the floor in front of you.

Slowly start to lift the outstretched leg as close to horizontal as possible. Don't worry if you can't get anywhere near horizontal to begin with. As your muscles strengthen, you will be able to lift your legs higher.
As the leg becomes higher, tense the whole thigh, and hold there for a few seconds (Picture 1)

Now, keeping the thigh horizontal, lower the calf, pivoting from the knee so that your heel swings under your thigh as far as you can go (Picture 2). It's a little like doing a Bicep Curl but for your thighs. This part of the exercise works the Bicep Femoris muscle at the rear of the thighs.

With any leg exercise, I prefer to aim for a higher number of repetitions.
Usually within the 20-30 repetitions. Once completed, switch over to the other
leg and repeat.
As this is a tough exercise you may only want to do 1 set for each leg.
Particularly if you are doing some squats in the same workout.

Exercise name: Jupiter Lunge
Benefits: Quadriceps (Large muscle on the front of the thighs) & Gluteus
Maximus (Muscles in the bottom)
Mindset: Great glutes. I know, I know, the ladies would love to have a great
butt and the guys like to look at a great ………. Let's leave it there shall we. I
think you know where the mind has to be.
In my opinion the best exercise for the buttocks is the lunge. In case you
haven't heard of this exercise. In its simplest form it involves taking one step
forward with one leg and with that forward leg lowering that leg into a squat
position with the other leg also being lowered until the second leg knee just
touches the floor as seen in picture on the following page.

The gluteus maximus are large strong muscles and therefore must be worked
hard, so don't be afraid to push yourself in this exercise. You may well find that
the quadriceps tire before your glutes but keep your mind on your ultimate
development.

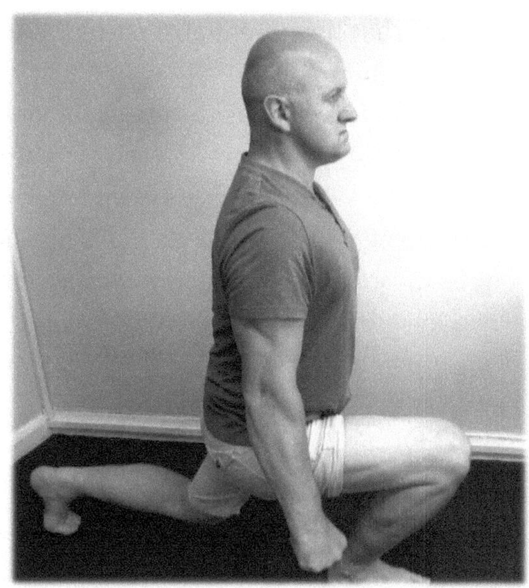

After raising yourself up switch legs and repeat.
The body will always remain in the same position.
Now, with the Jupiter Lunge it's a little different, in that you are going for a
slow walk whilst doing the lunge.

The exercise, for the first repetition is done as described above. When the first
leg is raised back to its starting position (let's suppose it is the right leg) instead
of standing still and then going down on the left leg. Take a step forward with
the left leg so that it is now in front of the right leg and complete the lunge.
Each movement should be done in a slow and deliberate manner. Concentrate
and feel the muscles being activated
It's a little like going for a walk but with each step being a lunge movement.
Balance may be a little difficult at first. If you wobble, simply stand back up to
the starting position and go again.

If the weather is fine, this is a great exercise to do in your back garden. Maybe
go round in a large circle and count how many circuits you can do. Have fun.
You may only be able to do a few Jupiter Lunges to begin with but after a short
time, this should build into a respectable number of repetitions and of course,
far firmer buttocks.

There you have 8 exercises that has the potential to change your entire physical appearance.
Put in the effort. Keep the tension on the muscles throughout each movement. Constantly strive for greater tension, concentration and increase in the number of repetitions and visualise about how you want to look.
If you want to adapt new movements and exercises that's fine. So long as there is continuous tension on the muscles throughout the movement then the muscles will adapt to what you are applying.

Congratulations. You have just Walked on Jupiter!

Now for the.................

The Body Weight Exercises:

So, if WOJ is so great, why have you included Body Weight Exercises?
Two reasons: -

1. Some people when exercising like to overcome a physical resistance and like to push themselves against a physical force. In this case body weight and gravity.

2. You can still apply WOJ principles when doing these exercises by slowing doing each repetition so that the resistance is greater because you are eliminating momentum.
Combine slowness of repetition, bodyweight and gravity and you have a serious workout ahead of you.

    Don't believe me. Quickly do 5 squats down and up, down, and up as fast as you can.
    Have a brief rest and now repeat but go down in 5 seconds and come up in 10 seconds.
    Can you do 5 repetitions?

Never knock Body weight Exercises. You don't have to have a dumbbell in your hand to build muscle. It's all about the resistance. Body weight Exercises work, period!

These are the basic exercises I would recommend, that cover most of all the major muscle groups.
As you are reading WOJ, I would recommend that you do them randomly, mix them up. Don't be a slave to a set system and format. Forget about religious exercise patterns. Go with what you feel comfortable with.
It's fine to mix up WOJ with Body Weight exercises. They are all beneficial.

Build things up as your body adapts to the exercises. If your body is tired a few days after working out, then please rest. It is better to rest more than exercise more if your body hasn't recovered.

The last thing you want is for your body to be in a continual fatigued state. This will only lead to a weak performance when exercising and can reduce the efficiency your immune system. Listen to your body.

Try and cover at least one of each exercise once or twice a week. This way it will give you an overall balance and stimulation to your body.

Some exercises you will enjoy more than others. Squats for example, people generally dislike because they are hard, especially when done slowly.
Please try and fit ALL the exercises into your routine. Even those you dislike. Think about the final destination, which is the new you.

Here they are:
Calf Raise on stairs.
Forward Squats
Upright squats
Press up
Kitchen Unit Dip
Extended Dip
Table Rowing

Seven exercises that will shape and transform your body. Don't worry if you have not heard of some of these before. They are basic movements, and some are just a variety on what you may have already done in the past.
I will go through each exercise with you and explain what parts of the body will be stimulated throughout each movement. I will also go a little in-depth about where your thinking should be, to help in your concentration and thus add benefits to each exercise.

Calf raises on Stairs:
Muscle group: Calves

Surprisingly a lot of exercise fanatics miss calf work out of their routine because they think of it as an unimportant body part. Maybe it's because your lower legs are far away from your eyes!
I've never heard a lady say, "Oh if only I could shape my calves." Problem is they are so wrapped up with the size of the thighs!
It's important to realise that the thighs only make up half the length of the leg. However, if you're a lady and you wear a skirt or dress, your calves are going to be on show. Believe me when I say that a good calf shape for men and women can transform the whole look of the leg.

Mind: Before you even start a single Calf Raise, think about how you want your legs and in particular your calves to look. Do you have that image in mind? If you don't, find one and concentrate on that image for around 30 seconds before you start the movement. This will tell your mind why you are doing this and will give you motivation and a final destination.

Physical: I have assumed that you do not live in a bungalow or a ground floor apartment. However, you can do this exercise equally well by either standing on the bottom step of your stairs, a step ladder, a block of wood or even an old-fashioned thick telephone directory.
With the front part of your feet resting on the edge of the step you should lightly hold on to the stair rail or if using a step ladder the sides of the ladder. With your feet together and legs locked, slowly raise your whole body until it is balanced on the tips of your toes. The upward movement should take around 3 seconds to complete. Once in that top position hold it for a further 2 seconds and then lower slowly until your feet are just past the parallel. Then repeat the movement for several repetitions until your calves have a real struggle to do one more repetition.

When you become stronger in your calves, you can try doing this exercise one leg at a time.

This is a random exercise that can be done at any time. So why not try going upstairs one calf raise at a time? Be imaginative and work those lower legs. The calves are a tough muscle to develop because we use them every day when we walk.

Persevere and you will attain a good calf shape. Always aim to do more reps each workout. Also, the slower the movement the harder it is and ultimately the better development.

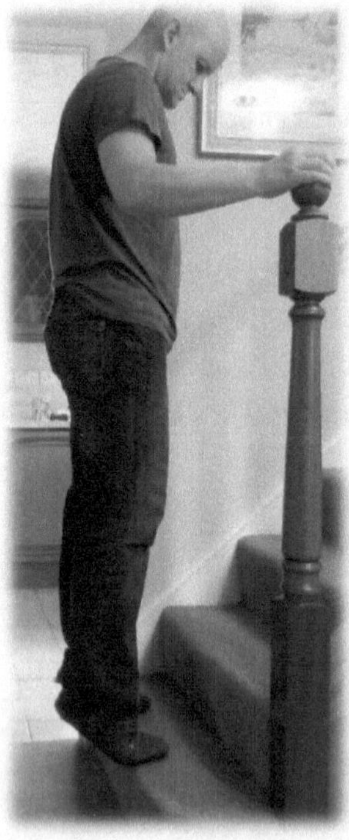

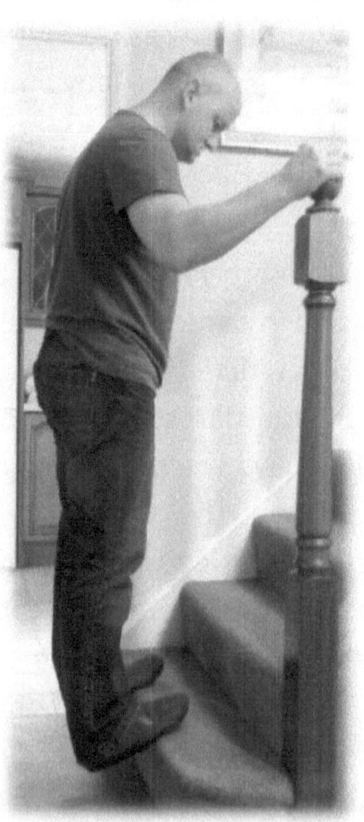

Elevated position   **Lowered position**

The Calf Raise is a simple exercise and can be done almost anywhere where there is step.

Try and get full range of movement and concentrate on the calves throughout.

When it gets easy to do around 20-30 reps then try doing it one leg at a time.

The calves are a stubborn muscle so persist and keep at it.

Very soon you will have added a new beauty and shape to the lower leg.

Forward Squats.
Muscle group: Predominantly hips and buttocks.

For most people squats are one of the most hated exercises out there. Why, because they're so tiring. You get exhausted quickly because of the lactic acid build up and you get a pain in your legs that can be pretty unbearable. So, to help you out with this exercise I am introducing you to the Forward Squat which is slightly easier than that of the Upright Squat.

Mind: This may well be easier for you ladies rather than you guys out there. Without sounding too sexist, the guys probably prefer to look at the Gluteus Maximus development of you ladies rather than being too bothered about their own!
Again, I want you to visualize that look of how you want to be. I know this area of the body is very personal, but you must have seen scores of pictures of models and film stars whom, if you are willing to admit, are slightly envious of. Well, if we're honest they didn't get that way by accident, I'm sure that just like you they had to work for it.
So, visualise (not idolise) away, get a picture of how you want to look before you start to workout
And know that change is on the way.

The exercise: This book on Exercise is for all people of all ages, to help them get into great shape and that is why I am going to offer you a variety of squat positions according to your current ability. If I was to start off with a full squat, then I may get complaints from people who could not get up again!
Initially however I am going to give you the exercise and assume that you are currently fit, strong and healthy and able to do a full range of a squat movement.

From a standing position with your feet approximately shoulder width apart and your arms out in front of you for balance, slowly lower your upper body until the backs of your thighs meet your calves. As you lower you may find that you automatically start to rise up on your toes. If this is the case you may want to start the squat with your heels placed on some books or a thin plank of wood.

You will also find that it is natural for the body to lean forward as you lower. This is okay as you are working more on the hips by doing so.

Balance may be a problem as you lower and rise, particularly at first until you get used to the movement and learn to balance. This can be overcome by gently leaning on an object in front of you such as a sofa, table, kitchen unit, dining chair etc. This is not cheating, it's just an aid for balancing.

A word of warning. Don't bounce as you come to the lower part of the squat. I know it's natural to bounce to aid you in getting back up again. However, this can be harmful to your knees, so lower and raise in a controlled fashion.

How many squats? Entirely up to you. If you've never done squats before you may find it difficult to do just one. That's okay, do one, have a brief rest then do one more. Build slowly.

Moving forward workout after workout is the key. Before long you will be doing lots of squatting before dropping!

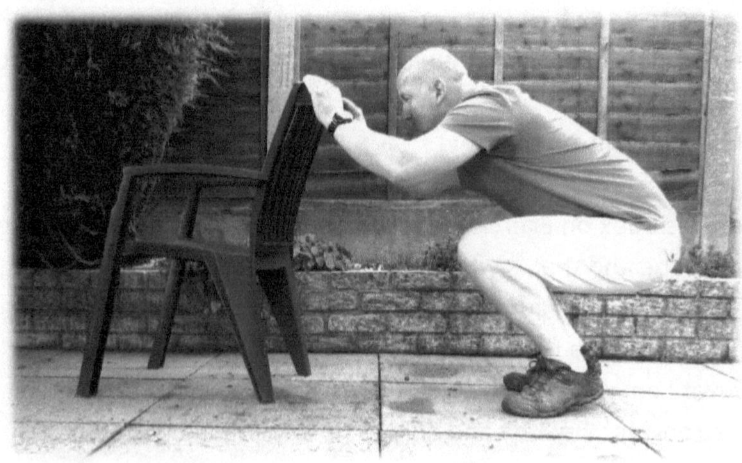

Leaning forward whilst doing the squat, makes it easier as you are putting more emphasis on the Gluteus Maximus (glutes) rather than on the thighs.
Always try and maintain good form with smooth movements to avoid any type of injury such as sprained muscles.
Feel free to support yourself on the back of a chair or something similar.

Ouch! I can't get all the way down, never mind back up.

Solution: Don't.

I fully appreciate that a lot of people reading this will have difficulty in going all the way down on the squat. This maybe an overweight issue, a knee problem, lack of flexibility etc. It doesn't really matter on the reason. However, you have to start where you are with what you've got.

May I suggest a chair? Preferably a firm chair such as a dining chair with four fixed legs but not an office swivel chair.

Now simply sit in the chair, lean slightly forward, look straight ahead, put your arms out in front of you and stand slowly. As soon as you are upright, lower yourself slowly back into the chair.

Keep repeating until you are tired out.

Keep repeating this for a few workouts and before long, you should be ready to disregard the chair. Build slowly, build safely

One more thing. Sorry about the muscle pain in the thighs and buttocks which you may well experience within 24-48 hours. This is natural, particularly if you are new to this exercise. This will ease over the next few days until you get used to squatting.

Upright Squats.

Muscle group: Predominantly Thighs and buttocks

These are done in a very similar way to the Forward Squats that I mentioned above. The exception being they are a lot harder as more emphasis is placed upon the thighs rather than the buttocks.

Mind: As this is primarily a thigh or upper leg exercise, that is where your concentration needs to be. Just like the buttocks mentioned above, I know you must have seen a great set of legs. If you're a man reading this, then I know you have! Seriously I know that you girls have too.

Wonderful thighs along with buttocks are probably the area that most women think about the most.

I've never heard a lady say, "Do my arms look big in this?" No, it always the bottom.

So once again take a few moments before exercising to visualise the look you want to have.

Exercise: Like the Forward Squat you can either stand flat footed or place your heels on a slightly raised object. You may also lightly hold on to something for additional balance if you desire.

However, this is where the difference to the Forward Squat takes place.

As you lower into the squat position keep the upper body vertical, keep looking ahead. When you are as low as you can go, return to the upright position, still keeping the back as vertical as you can. The slower you go the harder it is. I'm sure you will be aware of how much more intense and difficult this form of the squat actually is.

Some of you may find this movement too difficult to begin with. Please persevere and try and build up the number of repetitions.

As above, if you cannot do a single repetition then either go part way down and return or try lowering yourself to a sitting position on a chair and then rise. As the days and weeks go by try and increase the intensity as well as the number of repetitions and sets.

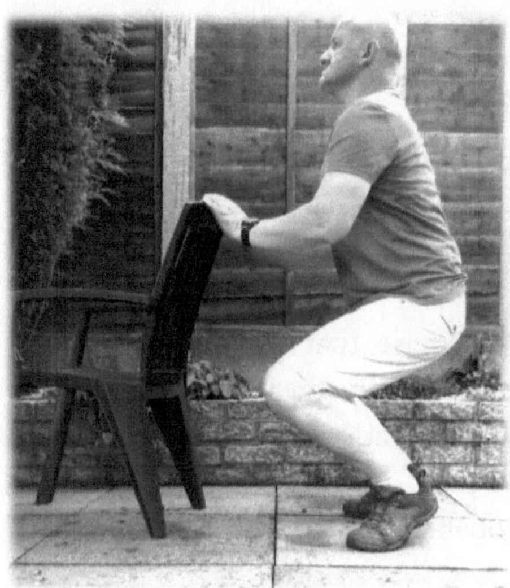

Picture (1)

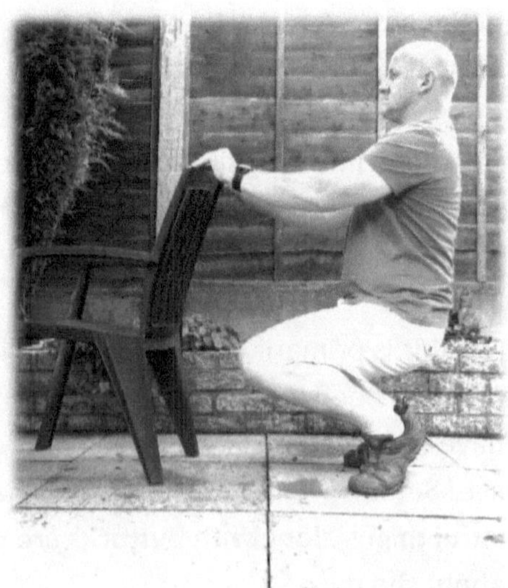

Picture (2)

As you raise into the upright position you will notice that I am still keeping my back straight throughout the entire range of the movement (see picture 2)
Also, the head is continually looking forward. It's important to keep the spine as straight as possible.
Intensity can be increased by NOT locking out the legs in the upper and lower final positions (see picture 1). This keeps continuous tension on the muscles.
Keep the back and the head straight. This will put a greater emphasis on the thigh muscles.
The slower that you return to the raised position the harder it is.
Continue to aim for greater intensity.
This exercise will cause a great increase in your breathing capacity. You may have to therefore rest at regular intervals even during just one set of Squats.

Press ups.
Muscle Group: Chest, Shoulders, Triceps, Abs, Thighs

You may be thinking, well what's so difficult about doing a Press Up. Most people know how to do this exercise. You simply get down, push your body up and down a few times, get up, job done.
I agree. That's it in its crudest form and some people like to do the Press Up as an ego boosting exercise. The more you do. the more macho you are!
However, if you truly want to master this exercise to get the ultimate benefit from it, then let's do it right. By doing so will certainly benefit your upper body. Primary muscle groups worked are chest, shoulders, and the backs of the arm. However, by tweaking this exercise, it can have the additional benefit of working the abs and thighs.

Mind: Time to visualise once again. As this exercise benefits the upper body, I want you to imagine what you will look like with toned shapely arms, broader shoulders, and a fuller more defined chest.
You should start to see yourself with separation between body parts rather than just a smooth overall appearance.
Visualise before you exercise. See before you be.

Exercise: I'm going to take you through the basic Press-Up movement and then offer you some varieties that will enhance other parts of your body.
Again, if you are unable to even do one Press-Up then I can help you with this until you become fitter and stronger and therefore able to get down and do the standard Press-Up.

It's worth pointing out that when do your first few repetitions you will be a little stiff and awkward. However, as blood flow starts to increase to the affected areas then it will become easier.
You may want to try just warming up by maybe doing just a few reps against a kitchen unit or on the arms of a chair for example. You are only half way down compared to a conventional Press-Up but it acts as a good warm up and makes the flow of the conventional Press-Up easier.

The basic Press-Up in its correct form should be done as follows: - Lie face down on the floor. Position your hands, palms down so that they are approximately shoulder width apart and just tucked under your shoulders. Let your body rise up slightly on your toes and now try and make your body as straight as possible.

At this point some people will try and make the exercise easier by arching the back to try and gain some leverage and momentum in raising up the body. Please try and avoid this and stick to good form even at the expense of extra reps. It is better to do 2 or 3 reps in good form rather than 10 reps with sloppy form. You're exercising your body not your ego.

Now rise. Push up using your arms to raise the body. Try and keep that body straight throughout the movement. Feel the muscles as they are being worked. Where do you feel that stimulation?

As you reach the top of the movement, tense your chest muscles for a moment before lowering.

At ground level try not to stop for an exaggerated length of time but try and push up and continue the flow of the movement.

When you feel you can't do any more, then rest for around 30 seconds on the floor and try and get maybe 2 or 3 more reps completed.

The idea is to try and go forward bit by bit, little by little, gain by gain.

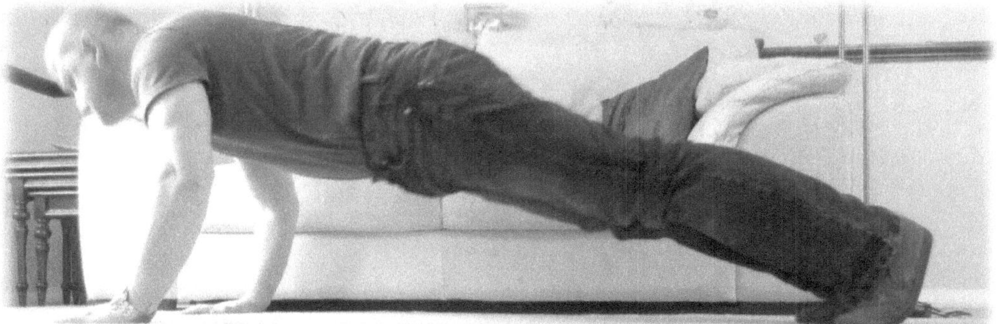

Notice the tension on the tricep muscles on the back on the arm. Aim to keep your body as straight as possible.

Focus your attention on the muscles being used and how you want your body to be.

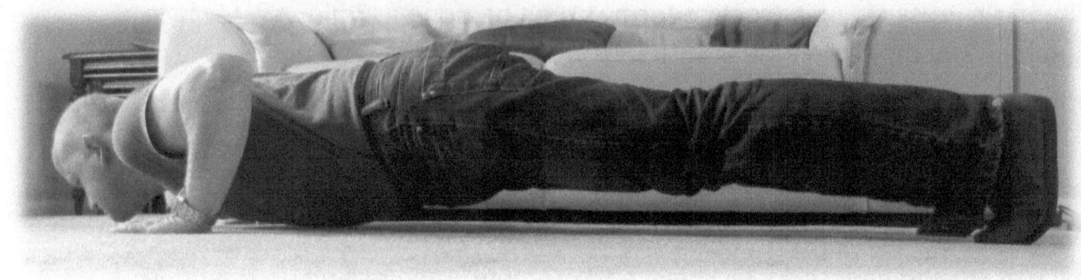

Aim to go all the way down, to gain maximum movement.
As you get to end of your strength limits, you could then maybe do partial reps
to push yourself nearer your potential.

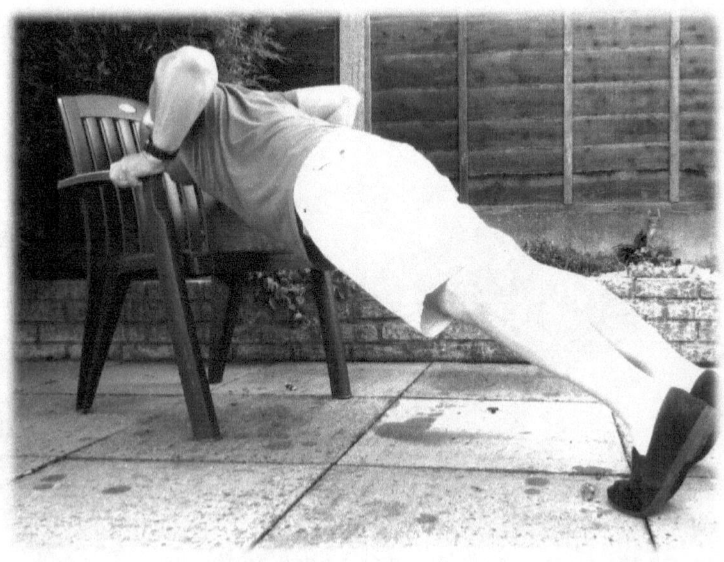

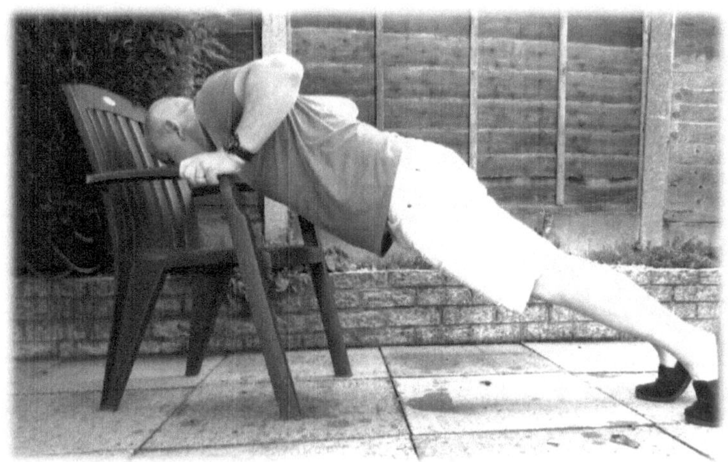

Yes, it is easier to do press ups when doing them with the aid of a garden chair or by leaning against a kitchen unit.
However, as I keep repeating it allows you a good range of movement and a good feel on the muscles being used.
The further the feet go back the greater the emphasis on the deltoids (shoulder muscles).

But I can't do a single Repetition! Yes, you can. Just do it differently. Try the following until you become proficient in the Press-Up. Don't feel guilty by doing this alternative style of Press-Up. Remember start where you are with what you've got.

I'm going to suggest 2 quick ways that can help you get started with the Press Up.

1/   Kneel down on the floor and then simply lean forward into the Press-Up Position. Your knees and lower legs will always be resting on the floor. Now with hand position as mentioned above, continue to do the exercise by pushing up on your arms. However, because you are not bearing as much weight on your Chest, shoulders, and arms, you will find it considerably easier. Build up until you can do the conventional Press-Up.

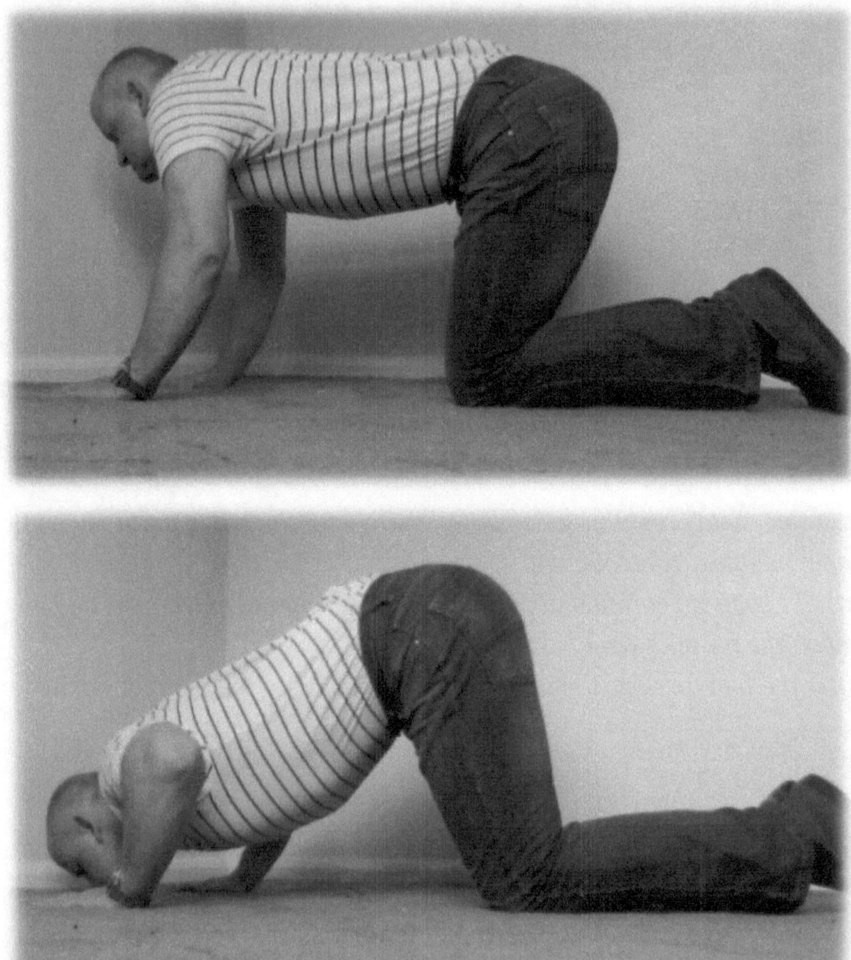

2/   Instead of starting the exercise from the floor in the horizontal position, try leaning against a kitchen unit or a similar piece of equipment such as a chair or the back of a sofa so that you are angled at around 30 degrees. Or you could try do Press-Ups by resting your hands on 2 chair seats positioned approximately 2 feet apart. These are not wimpy alternatives to the conventional Press-Up, just an aid to assist you until your body gets used to them.

Now onto some advanced form of Press-Up.
From the conventional Press-Up position place the hands together so that thumbs are touching. This will put more emphasis on the triceps muscles at the back of the arms.

Slow the exercise way down so that instead of coming up in one or 2 seconds, come up in around 5-8 seconds. This is so beneficial in that it puts total movement on the muscles rather than simple momentum.

Here's another variation: Instead of arms being shoulder width apart, place them further in front of you as though you are flying like superman. This is very difficult at first but as well as being a great shoulder developer, it also works the abdominal muscles as they have to support the whole body as it is stretched out.

Remember to concentrate and feel the muscles being worked.

Chair Dip.
Muscle Groups: Chest, Shoulders, Triceps

Sounds like a strange exercise. I have called it this as I simply do this exercise by using a couple of garden chairs. Also, it could be done by using your kitchen units if you have a 90-degree angle which many people will have allowing them to do dips. If you haven't, try using two dining room type chairs back-to-back around two feet apart. If using chairs, you may wish to put a towel over the backs of the chair to make it more comfortable on the hands.
Dips are an awesome exercise for the body. In fact, I would go as far as to say they are to the upper body what squats are to the lower body. They are just a great overall upper body developer.
Dips can be quite difficult for beginners; unlike the Press-Ups they involve you using your total body weight. However, don't worry if you can't do a single dip, as I will show you how to overcome this.

Mind: As this is an overall upper body developer, I ask you to imagine someone or even a group of people you admire in the way of upper body development.

Maybe for you ladies it is the person with the honed hourglass figure and maybe for you guys it's the man with the big strong muscular upper body, such as one of the action hero's you see at the movies.

I'm sure you already have someone in mind. Take a few moments out before starting the exercise to visualise how you will look.

Want an example of this. I came home from work and as I think back, I must have been 52 years of age when I did this.

It was around 8 o'clock. I normally finish work at my Engineering company around 5 o'clock. This night I had done around 3 hours extra. Normally I would make the excuse of, "I'm tired. I've worked over, I just need to chill." However, for some reason I was in the kitchen, not intending to exercise but instead I was flicking through You Tube channels on exercising. The more I saw, along with inspiring background music, the more I felt the urge to do a few Kitchen Unit Dips.

I started with feet on the floor as a warmup, but said to myself, I'll go for 10. Taking my feet off the floor, I lowered myself down. The first few reps were hard, and I concluded that I was because I was still a little stiff. However, I persevered and after 10, I did 12 and then 14. I thought that if I can get to 16 then I will have equalled my personal best from around 5 years previous! Well to my amazement I carried on and did 20 reps!

Well shocked, I was. I put it down to the mental preparation and inspiration beforehand. So maybe you can see now. Your exercise starts in your head and not in your body.

Exercise: As stated above this is a hard exercise, because of your total body weight being involved in the lift. I strongly recommend doing a warmup of this exercise by dipping but with feet on the floor so that when you raise, you are aiding the lifting by using both legs and upper arms.

Here's how. Stand either at the corner kitchen unit or between 2 chairs. Place your hands approximately shoulder width apart either on the unit or the backs of the chairs. In the upright position, slowly lower the body into the dipped position. Once there raise up the body by straightening the arms and legs. Try if you can by feeling the tension in the arms and chest. Tense your working muscles in the top position for 1-2 seconds and then lower to repeat the exercise.

Once warmed up, you can repeat the exercise with feet off the floor thus putting all the emphasis on the upper body.
Personally, I use both. I warm up with the feet on the floor, then rest a few moments. I then do as many dips as I can with feet off the floor, rest a few more moments then do what I can with feet back on the floor.

The beauty of this exercise is that if you have a relatively weak upper body then you can put more emphasis by lifting yourself with mainly legs until you become stronger.
You need to personalise this exercise to suit where you are currently at.

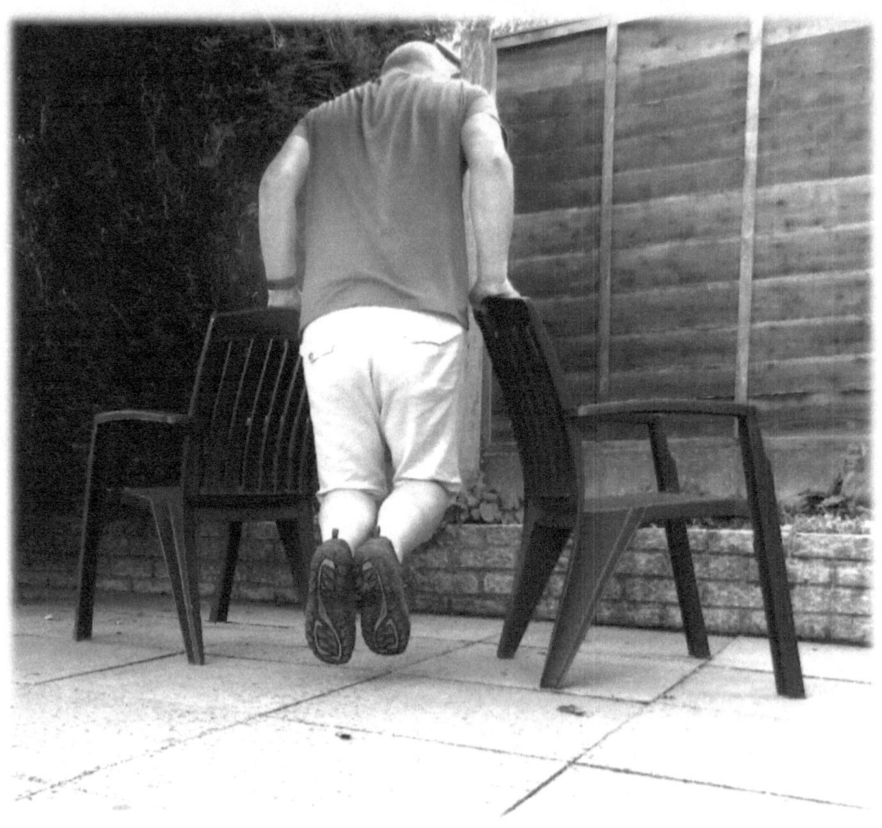

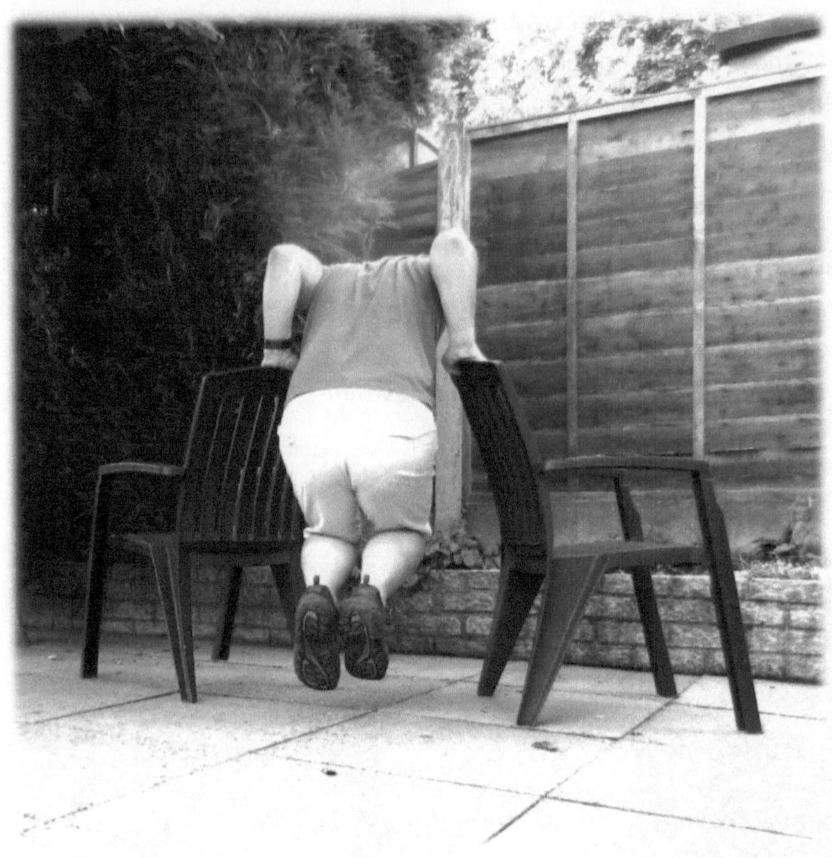

When dipping, try and keep the emphasis on the arms. Let them do the work. Try and keep the flow of the movement nice and smooth. This is a difficult exercise but can be made easier by keeping your feet on the floor.
(See picture on next page).
I tend to do it this way, not because I can't do normal dips but rather to allow me to feel the muscles being worked

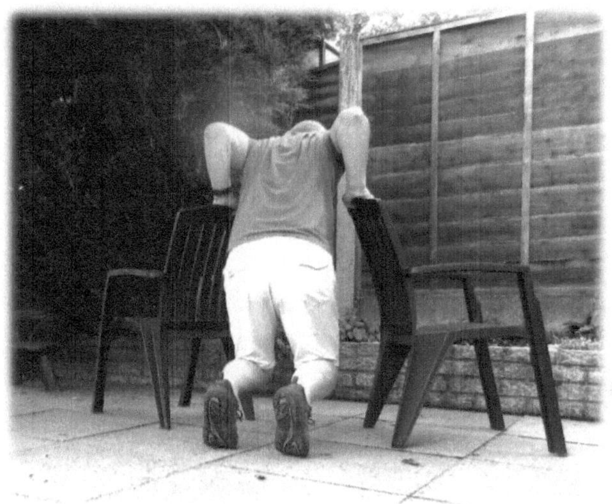

An easier way to Dip is with feet on the floor.

This is not a Wimps way of dipping but instead allows you to concentrate on the muscles being used.
It also offers greater flexibility, because as the arms tire, you can aid the upward movement by using your legs.

Extended Dip.
Muscle Groups: Chest, Shoulders, Triceps, Abs and Trapezius (upper back)

This is an awesome but often overlooked exercise. It's a little like the Dip mentioned above, but with your legs outstretched. I like to do this exercise in a slow and controlled manner as it is easier to concentrate on the muscles being exercised.
After just a few reps you will start to feel that soreness and ache in the abdominal muscles as well as in the Triceps.
You are also putting a greater emphasis on the back muscles particularly the Trapezius situated at the top of the back.

Mind: As above, this is primarily an upper body exercise, so that is where your concentration needs to be. See yourself with those shapely arms, firm upper body and well defined back.

Look at pictures of those people you admire. Spend a few moments concentrating and visualising on how you want to look.

Exercise: As with the Press Ups you have the option of either doing this in the parallel position using 2 chairs for example or at an angled position such as the kitchen unit. The more to upright you are the more difficult the exercise.

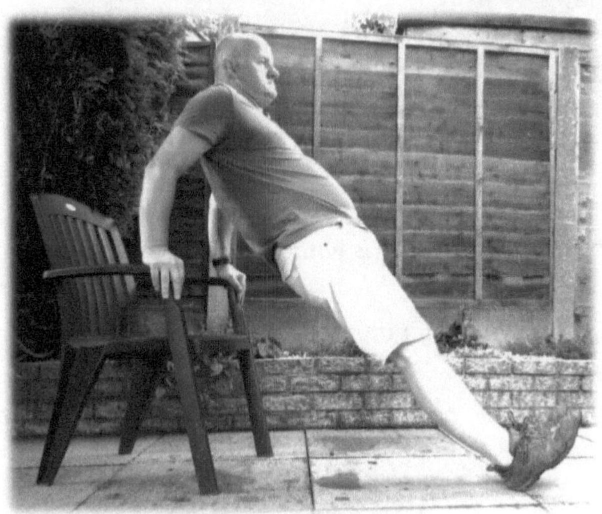

Picture (1)

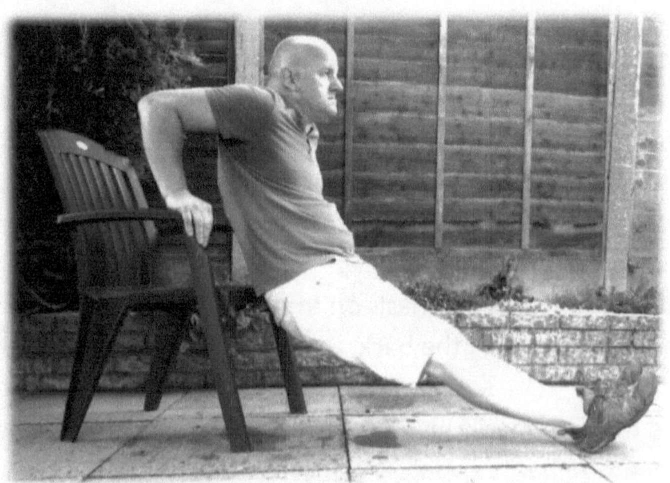

Picture (2)

As you lower try and keep your concentration on the muscles being used.
In this instance the triceps at the back of the arm, the upper back as well as the
tension that you feel on the abdominal muscles.

Again, I will take you through the process of the standard parallel extended
dip, and then on to the easier starting option of the angled extended dip.
Place 2 dining type chairs facing each other. How far apart depends upon your
leg length. Sit on the one chair and place your feet on the chair opposite.
Now place your hands palm down on the front edge of the seat so that they
are just underneath your bottom and thus should be around shoulder width
apart.
Now lift your body weight on your arms so that you are supported just with
your hands on one chair and the heel of your feet on the other.
Slowly lower yourself down so that your bottom nears the floor. When in the
fully contracted position, start to push up slowly by straightening your arms. As
you do this exercise you will note the tension in your triceps as well as a
tightening of the abdominal muscles as it tries to support the body.
As well as these muscles, you are also working the area of chest and upper
back. It really is a wonderful upper body exercise.

Now if that is proving too hard for you as a beginner to exercise, you can do
the above exercise but with your feet on the floor and your upper body leaning
either against the base of a chair or my old favourite the kitchen unit.
The nearer to vertical you become, the easier the exercise becomes. So again,
experiment until you find a starting position that is comfortable to you and
steadily extend the legs out, thus increasing the intensity of the exercise.

Table Rowing.
Muscle Groups: Sides of the back (Lats), Biceps, Forearms, Shoulders.

I have never seen this exercise done before. So maybe I am an inventor of a
new exercise, which I call table rowing.
The piece of equipment you will need for this is a solidly built table, or if you
don't have one of these, you can do this exercise with a good sturdy length of

dowel and two dining chairs placed around 3 feet or 1 metre apart. Place the dowel across the seats so it is firmly resting between the backrest and the seat. Doing it with the dining chairs is not unique, so I can't claim any fame for using that method!

This exercise is a sort of cross between doing chin-ups and using a rowing machine. This exercise will greatly stimulate the large muscles on either side of the back called the latissimus dori or lats for short. These muscles when developed offers that wonderful, "V" type shape to the back which looks great on both male and female alike.

Now, particularly you ladies, maybe saying, "So what about my back? I can't see what's behind me so I'm not going to bother about doing this exercise." This would be a mistake, as that lovely, "V" shape can be seen from the front as well as the back. Not only that, with the combination of the bicep, shoulder, and abs development that you also gain from this exercise, it can add a whole new and pleasing look to the upper body so please don't neglect this exercise.

Mind: I want you to think back; not reminisce about things you did in your past but think of your back and other people's great backs. Get inspiration from others. You often see the female film stars give a half turn when posing for photos. This is because it pulls the waist in and shows off a slightly broader shoulder and tapered back look to the upper body.

Maybe you could angle a couple of mirrors to see your back and then visualise the look you want to achieve.

Remember, visualise not idolise. You're you and you're special. You're great and you're going to get greater (hopefully humble as well). So put your back into it and enjoy this exercise.

Exercise: Take your average dining table or as indicated below an outdoor patio table.

I want you lie down under the table face up. Extend the hands forward and bring them onto the edge of the table. Now lift your body. It's a little like doing a press up in reverse. However, this is a pulling exercise rather than a pushing exercise. Again, you may find this exercise difficult to do at first, but with regular practice you will start to do many reps.

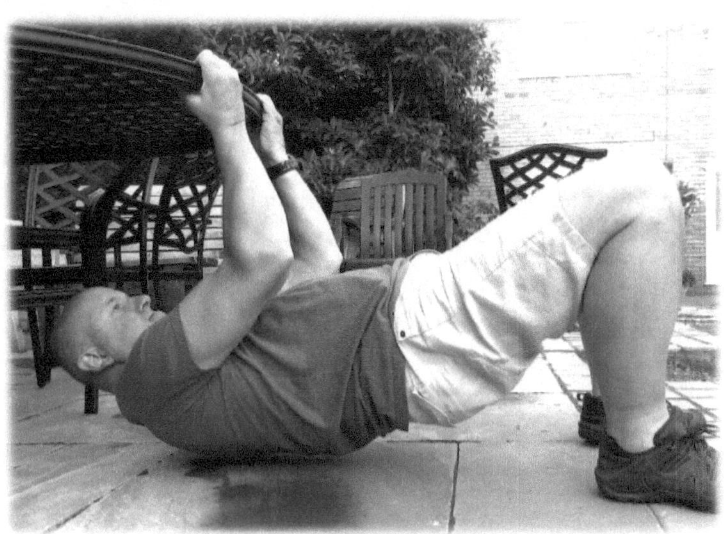

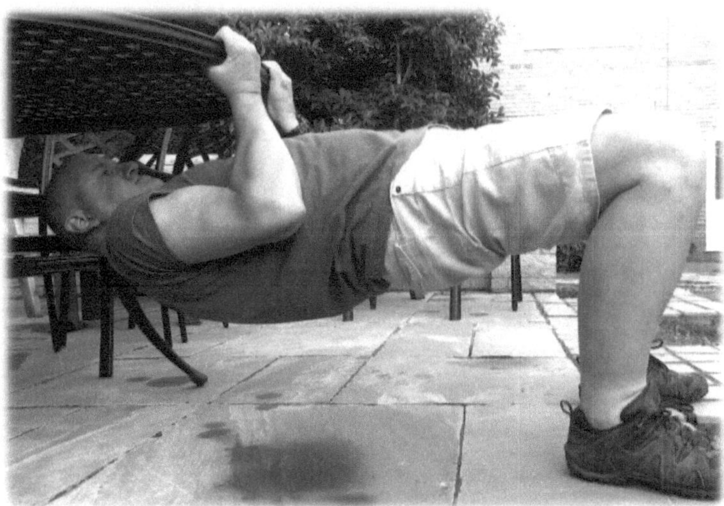

This is a tough exercise to do initially. However, if you persevere you will develop some shapely biceps and a pleasing back

I would also like to give you an easier option to begin with just in case you cannot do a single repetition.

In the position mentioned above, bring your legs back towards you so that you are in a lying squat position. Then pull up once again and you will find that your legs will be doing some of the work. As you progress, you can slowly extend the legs back out to make the exercise progressively more difficult.

Those seven exercises above are the basic building block exercises that I use on a regular basis. I don't do them in any particular order, and I don't generally do any more than 2 of the exercises a day. You may find that hard to believe, as most of what you have read will probably offer maybe 10 to 20 different exercise per session.

You may also find it interesting that I often have 2 or 3 rest days before I exercise again.

This means that I probably exercise around 30 minutes a week.

This means that I have could potentially have done a week's workout before you've even got to the gym and done your first repetition.

This means that in the past you may have dedicated around 2 hours, 3 times a week to getting changed, putting on your trainers, driving to the gym, parking, starting your routine, waiting for equipment, getting through (often enduring) your workout, getting back to your car, driving home, and flopping into bed because your exhausted through endurance.

This means you may spend between £200 and £300 per year for your gym membership plus fuel cost. However, most of what you need for your home workout is free.

This means in a year, you've not only spent a lot of money, but also time. In the above example around 300 hours in a year. That's 12. ½ days or nearly 2 weeks dedicated to getting to the gym to exercise.
Personally, I calculate my time to be around 62 hours in a year. That's around 2.1/2 days.

No excuses. I am sure that you can dedicate just 2.1/2 days in a year that will give you more confidence as you walk around in that new body for 365 days a year.

I asked the question at the beginning of this book: "Am I against gym workouts?" Absolutely not. Good gyms are full of state-of-the-art equipment. They're good places to socialise as well as work out. They often contain knowledgeable coaches and if the exercises are done correctly then you will see results. All I am saying is that they are not absolutely necessary.

In my early twenties I worked out in a gym and made some moderate progress. Problem was, I was stuck in the routine of obeying the exact number of sets and repetitions according to whose ever article I was reading!
However, I have to say that now in my sixties, working out using the WOJ method combined with those 7 exercises above and applying my mind to the workouts rather than just going through the motions have taken me to a whole new physical level.

Now what about that place we all love to be in. Can we really be……….

Working on Jupiter.

I think it certainly requires a mention. Hence this additional small chapter.

Can you work out at work in a discreet and almost stealth like manner and still get results, with the boss's permission of course?

As most people work an average of 8 hours a day, it kind of makes sense to try and include some body changing exercises whilst at work.

If we're being honest with ourselves, most people finish work, go home, eat their tea, watch tv and go to bed. If you mention any form of exercise, most people will say, "Forget it, I'm too tired, I've had a busy day, I just want to flop down on my sofa and chill out."

So, even though I'm going to get shouted down for even suggesting a workout in the workplace, I believe the little time it takes to do a few WOJ exercises can be vastly recompensed in the reward it offers to the individual as well as the company.

The people are paid to work not to exercise.

I fully agree, but before all you boss's out there kick off about this, it may be worthwhile looking at your absenteeism list to see who is actually away from your workplace due to physical or even stress related conditions. No; WOJ is not a cure all, but if your employees were healthier, happier, more energetic, and enthusiastic not only might they have less time off but may also work more efficiently whilst they are at work, thus benefiting the company as well as themselves.

So maybe taking a few moments in the day every now and then to do a just a few WOJ exercises may not be a bad thing after all.

A kind of win, win situation.

To be honest, Mr & Mrs Boss, you probably won't even notice your employees taking the time out to do the exercises anyway, as some of them appear to be simply stretching type movements.

It's all so simple. You don't have to get changed into any gym type outfit. You can do a lot of the exercises whilst sitting in an office chair or whilst squatting down to get something out of a cupboard.

Moving and tensing the body through the simple exercises actually increases blood flow and forces oxygen into the lungs thus giving you a more wide-awake experience.

That translates into less mistakes and improved productivity.

There's not a lot to lose by at least giving it a go. Who knows you could start a trend by being the fittest company in your area.

It works better if all are involved, this way you can inspire one another.

Motivation (although short lived) is a great way to spur each other on.

Invent new ways, new exercises, keep it fresh. The more physical and mental changes that are made, the more likely you are to continue working out.

Highlight the fact by putting it on the notice boards. Get copies of the book for the staff. Advertise the fact. It's new, it's different and it could be a great publicity campaign. After all, how many other companies are going to do this? Which leads quite nicely to the next question……………

What about the bigger picture?

We all want to be the one making a difference, so why not start a trend by transforming the workplace, the home, your neighbourhood and why not your wonderful nation.

Imagine the transformation if this country (United Kingdom) increased productivity by just 5% by WOJ and decreased the burden on the NHS by 5% through better physical and mental health.

What if absenteeism was to decrease by 5% and the joy factor in the workplace was to increase by 5% wouldn't we all benefit?

Personally, I love the UK, I believe it is a great country to live and work in. Small changes through exercise both physically and mentally can make a huge difference.

Why don't you be a part of it?

Now I've made an assumption as we come near the end of the book and ……..

I'm guessing that you still have questions:

Having read this far, you may still have questions? I don't know what you're going to ask, but here are some of the common ones.

Do I need to get the all clear from my doctor or physician before I start any exercise program?
Yes, I would highly recommend that you do. That way both you and your doctor will have peace of mind that you are up to it.

You say that you only do 2 exercises per day and then have 2 or 3 days off. How can this be right when most articles I have read state that you should exercise every day?
It really depends upon the exercise. Walking your dog in the park is exercise and that's great for you and the dog, and it will also make you a little fitter, particularly if you don't do any other exercise. However, it is not going to make much change to your overall body shape, unless you're vastly overweight and you walk a lot of miles and reduce your calories. Even when you lose the weight, you will probably be just a smaller version of you underneath. Not only that, because your muscle mass will not really have increased you will put back on any weight loss reasonable quickly.
If you want to re-shape your body, then you have to work up to working out hard. By doing the exercises I mentioned previously you will have to push yourself pretty much to the limit. Then do another set and maybe a third set if you have the energy and stamina. This will the force the body to make changes from the inside out.
However, because of the demands you have placed upon the body, it will take longer for the body to recover, hence going all out on just 2 exercises and then getting plenty of rest for the body to recover and change.

As I've stated many times in this book, all I can give you is advise and that advice is not set in stone. Please feel free to explore other methods of exercise.

How will I know when enough is enough?
Listen to your body. If you are new to the whole exercise thing, then initially I
would recommend that you don't push yourself too hard to begin with. Get
used to the exercises, visualise, and feel the movement. Don't jerk the body
into moving, this could cause a muscle pull or unwanted strain on the body,
and this could result in a lengthy lay off whilst you recover.
Follow the easy way of the exercises above and work up the work out.
The more you push yourself the greater the lactic acid build up and you will
reach a point when your body says that's it, enough. Stop.
Rest, and if you feel you can do another set then fine.
Remember too that the mind will always give out before the muscle.
The more you train, the more instinct will kick in and you will automatically
know when enough is enough.

I have my own favourite exercises. Can I use them instead of yours?
Of course you can. The exercises I recommend is what I consider to be good
all-round basic compound exercises. However, if you have your own, then use
them instead or in combination with my recommended exercises.
No matter what exercises you do I would suggest that you follow the principles
of visualising how you want to look and to feel the movement as you do it. This
is so that you can get the best out of each repetition.

Can I use weights or fitness equipment?
Again, I would have to say yes. If you really insist on lifting your dumbbells,
then lift. A great many people have sculptured some great physiques using
weights.
One of my many reasons for writing this was to simply say that you don't need
to go to a gym or fitness centre to get a great looking body. You can do WOJ or
body weight exercises almost any place at any time and in a fraction of the
time with no cost.

Added to this, some people are too embarrassed to go to the gym, because of
how they currently look. This book was written for those people as well as
anybody else who wants to get that awesome physique by working out
anywhere and at any time with minimal equipment.
My aim is to give you total flexibility.

Plateau's?

I'm glad I thought of that question! Plateaus are something that everyone goes through when exercising. This is generally how things work out: -

People go to the gym or exercise at home. Or maybe you will see the new enthusiastic jogger running along on the pavement. Within no time at all they are really pleased with themselves and are happy to tell you and the rest of the world that they lost 5 pounds in a week.

Come week two, and because they did so well in week one, they are inspired to keep on working out and sure enough they lose another 3 pounds. Great, well done.

The cycle continues and the third week they may lose a further 2 pounds and week four a further 1 pound.

Weeks five and six, just half a pound! All that work for half a pound! What's going wrong, I'm still working out just the same. In fact, I am running further, swimming further and playing more badminton and yet the weight is still the same. What's happening, apart from frustration?

It's called a plateau. You see your body will do everything in its power to stay the same.

If your body could speak, this is what it may be saying.

"Doing a lot of extra physical work. Danger! Danger! Must retain certain fat levels to provide energy for next exercise program. Therefore, keep fat on. Store as energy for next run."

Think about it. If your body constantly lost weight 24/7 then in next to no time you would die! Your body works on a sub conscious level. Without you thinking about it, it goes into survival mode and will adapt where necessary to keep your body working at an optimal level and that includes keeping certain fat levels. It's the way we were created to be.

Often you will see professional fitness models, or bodybuilders just prior to a photo shoot and they look awesome, like someone has come along and just scooped all the fat off their bodies.

Likelihood is that they have either been photoshopped to make them look good or they are genuine pictures, and they are now at the end of weeks of very hard training and dieting. See them a few weeks on and they will probably look quite different as they have probably gone back to normal eating patterns as a person's body cannot be starved of fat for too long.

It would be nice if our weight loss, and muscle gain was linear, but it's not.
Gains or losses, depending on who and what your body type is generally comes
in spurts.
This may help in................

Breaking the plateaus.
As I have previously said, your body craves normality. It loves to remain
constant.
In the early 1980's I attended a small gym. No free weights but just a few
pieces of weight training machines. For the first few weeks, I put on a bit
weight and muscle in the right places and then it stopped and remain stopped
for the next 3 years!
Despite reading countless articles from magazines and books I couldn't seem
to get past this over extended sticking point.
What finally did it was not more training but more resting. My body was
constantly tired and instead of giving it rest I was giving it more and more work
to do, whilst still exhausted on an inner level from the previous workout.

You don't know where your body is on a conscious level. You can't necessarily
say, yes, my body is fully recovered and here I go. If in doubt take that extra
day off from training and then go again.

Try changing things around. Break the normality mode. Do something new. As I
stated earlier I generally do just 2 exercises. However, when I do them, I will do
a set, rest, do another set rest. Then maybe have a cup of tea, watch a bit of
TV. Do some more in the commercial break. Do a few more maybe when I get
five minutes a couple of hours later. Go shopping, do a different exercise.
Maybe this time I have five to ten minutes to spare so I will do several sets in
this time frame which is enough time to push my body hard.
In other words, it's, "Totally Random." No getting changed into gym clothes.
No pre-work out drink, no equipment to set up. No waiting around. I just
visualise, get my mind right, get into the groove, do things slowly so as not to
pull a muscle, increase resistance, keep concentrating on the muscles being
worked and that's it.

I've achieved good results by doing just that, because my body doesn't know what's coming and when. It's in a constant state of surprise rather than set times, on set days with a set workout.

What else? You can try changing your diet. Have days when you just eat just salads. Maybe try a high protein day where you eat primarily meats so that your body gets the muscle building ingredients, it needs. If your brain isn't functioning as well as it should, or you're constantly lethargic it maybe that it needs more carbs, or you may need to drink more water.
I appreciate that your body needs a normal type of diet, but once every now and then try to supply it what you think it needs to help it fully recover and for you to be in that optimal state.
I may get shouted down for saying this, but also a have a food binge day. Sure, you may gain one or two pounds, but you will also be stocking the body up with all the nutrients it needs to make your next workout an optimal workout.

Yes, there's more.
The mind always controls the body. There's a saying, "Fake it, until you make it." I don't believe this is deceptive, but rather it's just asking you to visualise how you want to look. There is a verse in the bible which says." As a man thinketh in his heart, so he is." This is so true. You are where you are now because of your thoughts. Those thoughts have moulded you into the person you are today. Now do you think of yourself as fat and ugly because someone has told you that over and over again?
Maybe you've been ridiculed and unfortunately believed it to be true. You may have also added to it strong emotions. You now believe all that garbage and you've then told it to yourself over and over again thus reinforcing it.

Well now my friend it's time to break that habit.
Visualise, emotionalise, and verbalise, the person you must be, not want to be, not should be, but MUST be. A must is much stronger than a should or a want. Constantly see this in your mind. Look at pictures of how you must be. How will that feel when you look and feel and act as that new you. Talk out loud if possible. The car is a great place to shout things out. Get excited. Get energetic. You're brilliant. You can do it.

Do this and your workouts will change dramatically if you are in the right frame of mind. You can visualise better, you can go further with your number of reps. Your whole body and mind will get behind you in giving you your best performance and results.

Adopting the right mind set and physical actions can break a rut. Try it.

I've tried exercising before and it didn't work for me. Do I have a body type that doesn't respond to exercise?

No, you have an excuse that responds to, "I don't want to really try. Or what is the bare minimum I can get away with before justifying my lack of results?"

Agreed, as I mentioned previously there are different body types, and some will respond to exercise and body change far more rapidly than others.

However, please don't use this as an excuse. You can change.

If you have that body type that piles on the pounds just by looking at a lettuce, then try the following:

Eat less and more healthily.

As well as doing the aforementioned exercises, get out more. Walk with purpose, swim, dance, play. Just move about.

Constantly see before you, the sort of figure or body you want to have.

Nothing is impossible for you. If you believe it, you can achieve it.

DON'T continue to talk with your other fat friends about how much weight you've gained. I know I'm treading on thin ice here, but if you must socialise with people who are as out of shape as you might be now, then at least inspire each other to get into shape. Don't talk doom and gloom about how you are never going to get the body you want.

Exercise works. Period. So does a healthy diet. Set yourself a written goal. This will inspire you to work towards it.

Think about how you will react when your friends say to you, "Wow! What have you done to get into such great shape?"

I mentioned in an earlier chapter about adding muscle to the body. Whether you're male or female, it will give you a whole new look and better shape.

Added to this benefit is the fact that muscle increases your metabolism, which means that your body will burn off fat at a greater rate even when relaxing in an armchair. Providing of course you have put in the hard work beforehand.

Notice I said, the hard work. You must be willing to push yourself beyond your normal capabilities so that your body has a reason to change. Five Star Jumps is not going to do it!

I'm really hoping that you have read this far because I am now writing this next section around 18 months after typing the rest of the book.
A little secret that I use can have a great effect upon your muscular growth and shape.
Abbreviated it's PPFE," It's simply an acronym for, Pushing Past Facial Expression.
You're so cleverly designed that your body has certain, "Shut off," mechanisms built in so that you can only push yourself so far. One of those is a lactic acid build up in the body. When you exercise this lactic acid builds up in the area being exercised. For example, if you are doing squats after a short time your mind tells your body that's enough. This signal is reinforced by this lactic acid increase in the area of the thighs. This is the point where most people say. "That's it, I'm done." And stop the exercise.
The mind also adds to this by giving you a certain facial grimace that you see on athletes faces when they have just completed a marathon. It tells everyone around them that they have given it there best shot and look how tired I am.
So, let's take things to a new level by changing your face!
We'll use a set of squats as an example: -
You've got your mind right before hand. You've visualised the size, shape, and the look of how you would like your thighs to look like.
You start the squatting, in a nice even flow of up and down. You approach your mental target of 15 reps and your mind start to say that's enough. I'll allow you to get to 15 reps and no more. You've equalled your previous best and that's it. Be satisfied.
Your thighs are aching like crazy and you back it up with your face that is looking like it's chewing on a bag of nails. Everything within you says stop; beat your record number of squats next time. There's always tomorrow.
Remember what I said earlier about how the mind always quits before the body. Well, it just has.
Now try PPFE. This is where you have to be mentally aware of where you are during the exercise. When you reach that point of not going any further, I want

you to simply put you face straight as though nothing is happening and continue with your number of reps.

I have tried this many occasions and sometimes carried on doing a further 4 – 6 reps.

It's basically tricking your body into thinking that everything is okay because your face tells your brain that you have not yet reached maximum exertion. When you think you're at the end of your number of repetitions think again. This extra bit of effort can make the difference between success and failure. One warning; As this is a severe form of exercise, I would not recommend doing it every workout, as your body will need extra recovery time. Maybe just add this severe form of exertion occasionally.

Why don't you wear proper workout clothes?

Because you are reading, WOJ which is based upon doing random acts of exercise at random times. Here's one example of how it works out for me: - Our saucepans are kept in our lower kitchen cupboard. If I need to take out a saucepan, I have to squat down to take one out. Whilst I'm down there, in a split second I may, not every time, but I may decide to do a few squats. I will quickly visualise, and then exercise.

Doing a normal squat in this situation you would probably bend slightly forward and spring up quickly using momentum as an aid to help you in the lift. Bad on the knees and not that beneficial.

Personally, I would lightly hold onto the edge of the unit, with back straight and head up, come up very slowly in around 7-10 seconds. The difference is immense. Doing just a few of these takes around a minute. All is well so long as I don't forget to take out the saucepan on the last rep up!

Now back to the original question. If I was to go into normal proper workout mode according to the masses, I would say, "Now I am going take a saucepan out of the cupboard. At the same time, I will do a few squats. Therefore, before doing so, I need to change into my tracksuit bottoms, put on my gym vest, put on and tie up my trainers. Hopefully I won't get distracted whilst I'm upstairs getting changed."

This completely destroys the point of doing things spontaneously. In the time it takes to get changed you could have completed 2 or 3 sets of squats. Job done. Next workout is whenever I feel like it.

Doesn't that take some pressure off?

Unless you are wearing something totally inappropriate such as stilettoes, or a tight-fitting dress or trousers, then do the exercises spontaneously.

Often that spontaneity comes from something you may have just seen on TV or a conversation you've just had or maybe someone you've just seen and read about in a magazine. If you then feel compelled to do a mini workout, then go for it. Seize the moment.

Where are the Sit-Ups?

Simple; there aren't any. Do Sit-Ups if you want to. Personally, I believe that they are an overrated exercise. The benefits of doing hundreds of Sit-Ups is limited as the abs are only isolated at a small point during the movement. Did you know that it takes around 22,000 sit ups to lose just 1 pound of fat? Doing 30 sit ups a day it would take you 2 years to lose that one pound. No thanks!

If you want to do a direct ab exercise, then at least do crunches which are slightly more beneficial or leg raises as you keep your feet off the floor throughout the exercise.

Try doing the plank exercise. This is basically you keeping still whilst in the upright position of a Press Up but with your elbows on the floor.

After just a few seconds you will start to feel the burn in the abs.

But I can't see my abs!

If you adopt the above exercises, believe me they will come. You may not see them, because they're probably hidden by a layer of fat. Reduce the fat and they will appear.

How do I reduce the fat?

By training and adopting a sensible eating regime. There is no secret formula. If you burn or use up more calories than you are inputting, pure logic tells you that you will lose the excess weight.

I see people jogging everywhere. Surely if the masses do it, it must be the best way to lose weight?

I need to re-emphasise this point as you may not believe me. Let me use a friend of mine as an example. He's fit in that he can run a marathon. However, to look at him, you may think that his main exercise is pressing the button on the TV remote. Despite his hours of running, cycling and playing badminton he still carries a fair amount of body fat.

If you're overweight and you start to run, of course you will lose weight initially. However, after just a few weeks it's a catch 22! You run to burn fat, but your body needs to store fat to provide energy to run, so you end up with a stalemate situation in that your body more or less stays the same despite your greatest running efforts.

If you must run and I'm all for this method of running, try the following. It's called Interval Training and I read of one report that states it is a whopping 900% more beneficial than standard running.

This is how it works: -

1/   Put on your best jogging outfit.

2/   Slowly run for around 30 seconds.

3/   After that initial 30 seconds suddenly speed up to near maximum and do this for around 15-20 seconds.

4/   Revert back to a slow jog. After a further 30 seconds once again speed up to near maximum and do this for around 15-20 seconds.

6/   Revert back to a slow jog and repeat the process.

After about 5 minutes you will probably be pretty exhausted, which, if you're a runner is a lot shorter than your normal jogging time.

I know this is a little random, but if you have a short 5-10 minute time slot give this a go twice a week. Try it for a month and see the difference.

Do I need supplements and protein powders?

It's all in the name, "Supplements." This means that they are a supplement to or are an addition to your normal diet, but they do not replace a normal diet. If you eat reasonably healthy most of the time and therefore include lots of fruit and vegetables in your diet, you shouldn't need extra pills and potions as the food you eat should contain all the nourishment you need.

We hear and read about professional Body Builders taking buckets loads of various supplements, including amino acids and various protein drinks. I know their picture and comments are next to a plastic container of powder or pills, and they may well take them. However, remember that being a professional, means that they get paid for being a professional. They may well use what they endorse and it maybe because they must be at their peak, particularly before a contest because their careers are dependent upon them getting a top position in the competition.

For the 99.9% of everybody else we will probably never push our bodies to the extent that they do or spend huge amounts of time in the gym.

To stress once again, a healthy balanced diet should give your body what it needs.

If you feel you must take something extra, then for the vast majority of people a good multi-vitamin / mineral tablet once a day should keep your body topped up with the nutrients it needs.

Can you tell me again how must rest I need?

This is very difficult to ascertain as everyone is different. A fit teenager for example may have loads of energy and feel that they could work out all day, every day. Probably not a good idea, but I know where they're coming from.

I sometimes have days where I feel super energised, and I may exercise 2 or 3 days in a row. I know this is contrary to what I stated previously. This is rare, but if I feel like going for it then I go for it. Remember, no rules.

A sluggish overweight person in their fifties probably feels tired whilst walking to the kitchen. To them this it is a super intensive workout as this is where the doughnuts are kept!

You need to have rest. After an effective workout your body needs to rebuild from the punishment you have just given it. Workout again too soon and your body will go into downward spiral mode, and you start getting into a rut.

You may start to feel tired and sluggish and develop minor illness's such as having a cold as your body starts fighting back. In other words, it's telling you to STOP exercising and recover. Please, listen to your body.

My muscles are so sore the next day. Is this normal?
Yes, very normal, particularly if you have worked out reasonably hard for the first time. I recently showed some people how I did some of my leg exercises in the back garden on a hot summers evening. They copied what I did for about five minutes, and we had some good laughs along the way.
They didn't think too much of it until the next day when then their legs just ached liked crazy. They couldn't believe how much muscle soreness there was after just a few minutes of exercise.
This is just simply because you have asked your body to do something out of its comfort zone. They may ache a few more times after this, but very soon your body will get used to it and the soreness will stop.

Build things up slowly and increase the duration and intensity as you go along.

So let's bring everything together for the…………..

Conclusion:

I really want to congratulate you if you have read this far. The vast majority of people won't have done so and may have already dropped out of doing the exercises. If they ever began!
I also hope that you have enjoyed reading and applying at least some of the contents of this book. If you have, then changes will start to take place.

As with anything new the difficult part is starting. Think of a rocket launch into outer space. Huge amounts of fuel are required to provide boost to propel the rocket up and through the earth's atmosphere. Once there, far less energy is required as the rocket doesn't have to escape the earth's gravitational pull. Motivation, energy, and the will to do it can be extremely difficult, especially at the start where little of no results can be seen.
However, once in the flow, your mind and body will get used to the new routine and things will get easier.

You see the majority of people who have read this will just simply go back to the way they were without really giving it a go.
They may pick and prod at the content of the book stating that it's not real exercise, or it's fake and not really hardcore gym workout and I appreciate that everyone is entitled to their opinion.
How you react to this book is entirely up to you. All I ask that if you are serious about body change then change your thinking from old school and at least give it a go.

People generally take the path of least resistance and go back to how they were and start blaming everyone except themselves for the way things turn out.
I really hope that you are not that person. Only you are responsible for you.

This may well be the end of the book, but it may also be your new beginning. If you adhere to what you have just read, you will change inside and out.
Remember that your life is a journey, enjoy it and live life to the full. It's not how you start this life; it's how you finish it.

Irrespective of age, each day is a new day for all of us. How you spend it, is up to you. If you think right, talk right, act right, eat right, and exercise right then the only limitations you have is what you have given yourself. Change your mind and you change your life.

Never blame anyone else for your outcome. Life will throw some tough stuff at you. It's not the stuff that bad. That's only a situation or circumstance. Rather it's how you react and then act. The more you overcome, the more you become.
Remember you have self- control so don't let anyone control you.

Work hard, have fun, don't resist change if it's for your good and live your new life to the full starting today.

One final thought. If you want to contact me or share how this book has helped you then please feel free to contact me at: andyelliott62@gmail.com
I will do my best to respond as soon as possible.

Any information will not be shared unless I first have your permission.

Finally, finally. Whilst writing this book, I think I became a little obsessed with using the word, "However." I used it 78 times!
Sorry about that.

God bless you.
Andy Elliott.

Goals:-

Use this section to write down, visualise, and even cut out and stick inspiring pictures of how you want to be.

Write down before and after measurements and body weight.

Turn to this section continually as an inspiration and motivation to continue pushing yourself forward.

Goals:-